TSONGKHAPA'S
Six Yogas of Naropa

TSONGKHAPA'S
Six Yogas *of* Naropa

by
Tsongkhapa Lobzang Drakpa

Translated, edited and introduced by
Glenn H. Mullin

Snow Lion Publications
Ithaca, New York

Snow Lion Publications
P.O. Box 6483
Ithaca, New York 14851 USA
tel. 607-273-8519

Illustrations by Christopher Banigan
Illustrations copyright © 1996 Snow Lion Publications

First Edition USA 1996

Printed in USA

ISBN 1-55939-058-1

Library of Congress Cataloging-in-Publication Data

Tsoṅ-kha-pa Blo-bzaṅ-grags-pa. 1357-1419.
  [Zab lam Nā-ro'i chos drug gi sgo nas 'khrid pa'i rim pa yid ches gsum
ldan źes bya ba. English]
  Tsongkhapa's Six Yogas of Naropa / Tsongkhapa Lobzang Drakpa ; trans-
lated, edited and introduced by Glenn H. Mullin.
    p. cm.
  Includes bibliographical references.
  ISBN 1-55939-058-1
  1. Nāḍapāda. 2. Yoga (Tantric Buddhism)--Early works to 1800. 1. Mullin,
Glenn H.   II. Title.
  BQ7950.N347T79 1996
  294.3'443--dc20   96-6980
                                                                              CIP

---

*This book is only for those who have
received a highest yoga tantra initiation.*

Table of Contents

A Book of Three Inspirations: A Treatise on the Stages of Training in the Profound Path of Naro's Six Dharmas by Tsongkhapa Lobzang Drakpa

Dedicated to the late Italian monk Stephano Piovella,
and the late British monk Kevin Rigby,
both very dear friends on the path to enlightenment,
and both of whom made great efforts to fulfill
the visions of the buddhas and bodhisattvas.
May they pick up in future incarnations
from where they left off in this,
and catch the wave of meritorious energies
everywhere surging since time without beginning.

Preface

Anyone who has read more than a few books on Tibetan Buddhism will have encountered a reference to the *Naro Choe Druk* (Tib. *na ro'i chos drug*), a phrase that renders literally as "Naro's Six Dharmas," but is more often encountered in English translation as "the Six Yogas of Naropa." These six—inner heat, illusory body, clear light, consciousness transference, forceful projection, and the *bardo* yoga—represent one of the most popular Tibetan Buddhist presentations of yogic technology to come from India to the Land of Snows.

The Tibetan word *choe* (Tib. *chos*) in the expression *Naro Choe Druk* is a translation of the Sanskrit term *dharma*, which means "doctrine," "teaching," "instruction" or "yogic training." *Druk* means "six." Thus the system can be called Six Dharmas, Six Doctrines, or Six Yogas. I generally use "the Six Yogas of Naropa," or simply "the Six Yogas," because these are the forms best known to Western readers. Occasionally I resort to the more literal "Naro's Six Dharmas," although whenever I do so I enclose the phrase in quotation marks in order to indicate that I am honoring the Tibetan form of the name, *Naro Choe Druk*.

Tibetan literature randomly refers to the illustrious Indian Buddhist master after whom this tradition is named as Naro, Naropa, and Naropada (born 1016). Naropa was a disciple of the Indian mahasiddha Tilopa (b. 988). The lineages that Naropa gave to his Tibetan lay-disciple Marpa Lotsawa (lit. "Marpa Translator"; b. 1012), especially that of the Six Yogas, came to pervade thousands of monasteries and hermitages throughout Central Asia, regardless of sect. This is certainly true within all the *Sarmai Choeluk*, or "New Schools," such as the Kadampa, Kargyupa, Sakyapa, Jonangpa and Gelukpa. In addition, the Six Yogas have also gradually become absorbed into most of the *Nyingma Choeluk*, or "Older Schools."

The treatise on the system written by Tsongkhapa the Great (1357-1419)—*A Book of Three Inspirations: A Treatise on the Stages of Training in the Profound Path of Naro's Six Dharmas*—is regarded as one of the finest on the subject to come out of the Land of Snows. Lama Tsongkhapa was the forefather of the Gelukpa school (Tib. dGe lugs; lit. "Order of Excellence"), which quickly swept across Central Asia and became the largest single school of tantric Buddhism. He was also the guru of the First Dalai Lama (b. 1391). His treatise has served as the fundamental guide to the system of the Six Yogas of Naropa as practiced in the more than three thousand Gelukpa monasteries, nunneries and hermitages across Central Asia over the past five-and-a-half centuries.

The Gelukpa lineage came down over the generations to the present day. The principal transmission holder, when I arrived in India in 1972, was Kyabjey Trijang Rinpochey, the Junior Tutor of His Holiness the Dalai Lama. He in turn passed it to numerous disciples.

I was in Dharamsala in 1973 when Kyabjey Rinpochey delivered his last transmission on Naropa's Six Yogas. At the time I was studying Tibetan language, philosophy and meditation at the Buddhist Studies Program initiated by H. H. the Dalai Lama as part of the activities of his recently established Library of Tibetan Works and Archives in Dharamsala. A few months into the program it was announced that the Junior Tutor to His Holiness, the very venerable and very elderly Kyabjey Trijang Rinpochey, would be giving a teaching in the museum room, the largest space in the building. The subject would be the Six Yogas of Naropa, and the recipients would be a large group of Tibetan yogis, hermits, monks and nuns. We Westerners couldn't attend, but if we liked we could sit in an adjoining room and listen through the sound system.

The Dalai Lama's Junior Tutor was considered to be one of the greatest living masters to come out of Tibet, and was regarded as a living buddha by the Tibetan community. News of his discourse had travelled throughout the refugee communities of India and Nepal, and great lamas began to roll into town from all directions. One monk who was pointed out to me was said to have spent more than forty years in meditation in the mountains. There were dozens of others with twenty or more years of solitary retreat under their belts.

Rinpochey spoke six hours a day for many, many days, using the text of Lama Tsongkhapa as his focus. One day one of the yogis coming out of the room at the end of a session looked at me and said, "Really, what a buddha he is!"

When this great lama passed away a few years later, the Tibetan spiritual community mourned the loss of one of the last of the supergreats to come out of Tibet. When I think back twenty-two years ago to the faces in the front couple of rows at that teaching, many of them have today come to rank among the foremost lamas in the Gelukpa school.

Essentially there are two main ways to teach Tsongkhapa's *A Book of Three Inspirations*: by means of a *shey tri* (Tib. *bshad 'khrid*), or "explanatory discourse"; and by means of a *nyam tri* (Tib. *nyams 'khrid*), or "experiential discourse." The former is what is most often received first. Usually this kind of teaching is given by a senior lama at a large public gathering, and entails a word-for-word reading and explanation of the text. The discourse of Kyabjey Trijang Rinpochey belongs to this latter category, as does the teaching I received from His Holiness the Dalai Lama in 1990.

Those who have attended a public teaching of the text and want to pursue the training will arrange to receive the second type of teaching, the "experiential discourse," which is given more privately. Here all philosophical and historical discussions are set aside, and the focus instead is placed on the actual yogic and meditative applications. This was the teaching style in Gelukpa practice hermitages; the resident teacher would impart a few pages of the text, and the disciples would then meditate for a few weeks or months on the material that had been covered. Only when the teacher felt that the desired inner experiences had been generated would he teach the next section of the text. Most practitioners receiving an "experiential teaching" of the text from their personal lama would already have received the "explanatory teaching," together with the appropriate empowerments, from a senior lineage lama.

Tsongkhapa's treatise was published in English—in an edition riddled with hundreds of errors—by Dr. C. A. Muses and Garma C. C. Chang in 1961 (*Esoteric Teachings of the Tibetan Tantras*, Falcon Wing's Press, 1961). Because the treatise itself is of considerable importance, the editorial staff at Snow Lion Publications felt it imperative that a more accurate rendition be prepared. They approached me with the request to accept responsibility for the project.

To prepare the first draft, I listened through the tapes of a reading of Tsongkhapa's text given by His Holiness the Dalai Lama in Dharamsala in 1990, which I had had the good fortune to attend. Although this was a wonderful teaching, it was of limited value for translation purposes, as it was not a "word-for-word commentary" (Tib. *tshig 'khrid*), but rather was a "meaning commentary" (Tib. *don 'khrid*). Therefore I undertook a private reading of the text with Geshey Lobzang Tenpa of Ganden Shartsey Monastery, who at the time was residing at Kopan Monastery in the Kathmandu Valley, Nepal. Later one of my root gurus, Ven. Doboom Tulku, kindly made time in his busy schedule to fly up from Delhi to Kathmandu in order to help me check my translation, and we were able to complete two-thirds of the work, up to the end of the section introducing the general principles of the illusory body and clear light doctrines. A few weeks later I had the good fortune of meeting up with another dear lama friend, Ven. Ngawang Pendey of Drepung Loseling Monastery, and he consented to help me check over the remaining third of the manuscript.

In addition, with Ngawang Pendey I read through several other treatises on the Six Yogas system, including the shorter of the two texts on "Naro's Six Dharmas" found in Tsongkhapa the Great's "Collected Works" (Tib. *gSung 'bum*); this is his *Mikrim* (Tib. *dMigs rim*), or "Stages of Meditation," which I plan to include in a forthcoming collection of readings on the Six Yogas of Naropa. With Ngawang Pendey I also read through several short commentaries on Tsongkhapa's *A Book of Three Inspirations*, including those by Gyalwa Wensapa (b. 1505), Ngulchu Dharmabhadra (b. 1772), and Jey Sherab Gyatso (b. 1803); I have drawn extensively from these in the introduction and notes. Later I re-checked several sections of these various works with Geshey Lobzang Tenzin, also of Drepung Loseling. Finally, some months later when I was back in Canada I had the honor of meeting up with another very dear lama friend, Zasep Tulku Rinpochey of Sera Jey Monastery, and at his Ganden Choling Meditation Center in Toronto checked through a number of passages regarding which I still had points of doubt, including the Epilogue and the section dealing with the physical exercises, which is written in a rather cryptic form.

The actual work of translation began quite auspiciously in Lhasa, where I was leading a group from the Tampa Art Museum, Florida, on pilgrimage to the holy places of Tibet. The bulk of the writing took place in my home-away-from-home, Room 405 of the Snow Lion Guest House, Chettrapati, Kathmandu, with its window looking up at the holy Swayambu Stupa. For me, setting is important to the task of setting pen to paper. Although the Kathmandu Valley has become somewhat chaotic and polluted over the past decade due to the tremendous influx of mountain villagers, the aura of sacredness emanating from its many holy Buddhist sites still shines with great strength. Preparation of the final manuscript was done at the country cottage of a New York friend, Ms. Lulu Hamlin, who over the years has greatly encouraged and supported my Dharma activities. Prof. Alex Wayman of Columbia University kindly offered guidance on technical matters, and Jimmy Apple of the University of Wisconsin generously helped in tracing down the many scriptural quotations that ornament Tsongkhapa's treatise. Over the year that the writing took place a number of other friends also helped with various details of the work; in this regard I would especially like to thank Conrad Richter, Michael Robillard, Pierre Robillard, Atisha Mullin, Hilary Shearman, Heidi Strong, Tina Teno, Athena Tara, and Debby Spencer. Finally, the staff at Snow Lion—Sidney Piburn, Susan Kyser and Jeff Cox—offered much valuable advice and support.

Fifteen years ago in a conversation with a very dear spiritual friend, Lama Zopa Rinpochey of Kopan Monastery, Nepal, the topic of translating tantric scriptures for open publication came up. I replied that I was somewhat hesitant to work with tantric material because of the self-professed secret nature of the tradition. Rinpochey laughed and replied, "When we came out of Tibet we all thought of the words of tantra as secret. But actually they are really self-secret. You should translate and publish tantric texts. It could benefit people. Those without a connection won't buy the book; or even if they do, they won't be able to understand the meaning."

I remember once when I was living in Dharamsala a friend's father came to visit. He picked up a book from the table, opened it at random, and began to read it aloud. The chapter was on the topic of the logic of emptiness. After a page or so he looked up, a somewhat stunned expression on his face, and said, "You know, there was not a single word on that page that I didn't know. But I don't have a clue what the thing as a whole is talking about."

On the other hand, when one approaches self-secret literature in its own environment, allowing it to speak in its own words and to use its own metaphors and illustrations, a sense of the profound integrity of the language soon begins to dawn.

Throughout the text the names of the Tibetan masters who are quoted or referred to are spelled simply as they sound in English, i.e., *Jey Sherab Gyatso* rather than *rJe shes rab rgya mtsho*. For the specialist, these are given in their transliterated forms in the glossary. In the main body of the text I do not use diacritical marks on Sanskrit names and terms, as these are distracting to the general reader; but again they can be found in the glossary.

As is standard practice with classical Tibetan authors, Tsongkhapa quotes all Indian texts from their translated versions preserved in the Tibetan canons, and gives the titles only in abbreviated Tibetan forms. Hence he will refer to the *Shri samputa tantra raja tika amnaya manjari* simply as *Manngak Nyema* (Tib. *Man ngag snye ma*), which in Sanskrit would become *Amnaya manjari*. Similarly, Tibetan textual titles appear only in condensed forms. I have followed a policy of giving all titles in English translation wherever this seems practical, followed at their first occurrence by the abbreviated Sanskrit or Tibetan forms in parentheses. Again, here diacritics are not put on the Sanskrit, but all texts are listed in the bibliography with fuller forms of both the Sanskrit and Tibetan titles of the Indian works.

I have done my best to insure that the translation is error-free; but Tsongkhapa's text is profound, and no doubt some hazy readings have found their way into the fabric of my work. Here I can only echo the sentiment expressed by Tsongkhapa in a closing verse of *A Book of Three Inspirations*, in which he addresses the subject of his concern with any errors that he himself may have brought into his composition:

> The essence of the profound teachings is hard to perceive
> And ordinary beings cannot easily penetrate them.
> Hence I request the *dakas* and *dakinis*
> To be patient with any faults of my treatise.

As Tsongkhapa states again and again in *A Book of Three Inspirations*, an understanding of the context of the Six Yogas, and thus an appreciation of its profundity, is greatly facilitated by an understanding of the Guhyasamaja Tantra system known as the *Five Stages* (Skt. *Pancha krama*). Unfortunately none of Tsongkhapa's quintessential Guhyasamaja material has yet been translated. This is the next big step in the transmission of the Gelukpa tantric system.

The tradition of "Naro's Six Dharmas" has fascinated and delighted Central Asians for almost a thousand years now. As Tibetan Buddhist studies continue to mature in the West, it will undoubtedly also receive considerable attention here. If this work can make a small contribution to the understanding of this extraordinary legacy, my purpose in undertaking the project will have been fulfilled.

Glenn H. Mullin
Snow Lion Guest House
Chetrapatti, Kathmandu, Nepal
March 14, 1995

Introduction

TSONGKHAPA AND THE LINEAGE OF THE SIX YOGAS

Tsongkhapa the Great stands as a colossal figure in Tibetan spiritual history. One of the most creative of the many illustrious writers, philosophers and scholar-yogis to grace the Land of Snows, he is usually referred to in traditional literature simply as *Tsongkhapa Chenpo*, "Tsongkhapa the Great," or as *Gyalwa Nyipa*, "the Second Buddha." His *Collected Works* reveal the depth and scope of his endeavors, which encompass the entire range of Buddhist thought, both in the *Sutrayana*, or public teachings, and the *Mantrayana*, or esoteric tantric doctrines.

His appearance on the Tibetan scene was timely. Less than two centuries had passed since the Turkic invasions of India had destroyed Buddhism in the land of its birth. Yet long before the destruction was complete, Tibet had absorbed much of what had existed in Buddhist India. The threads of the diverse lineages were scattered across the vast Central Asian plateau, to be found in mountain hermitages, monasteries, cave retreats and other sites of spiritual activity.

The spread of Buddhism in Tibet is usually divided into two periods: the Early and the Later Disseminations of the Doctrine. The first of these refers to the transmissions that occurred prior to the end of the tenth century C.E.; the second refers to the renaissance of the eleventh century, and the plethora of schools and sub-schools that this spawned. The Six Yogas of Naropa belongs to the period of the Later Dissemination of the Doctrine.

Tibetan records of the influx of Buddhist teachings do not provide us with much detail on the period prior to the seventh century. However, in approximately 650 C.E., under the rule of King Songtsen

Gampo, Buddhism became the country's national religion. From this time on, the importation of Buddhist lineages was systematically executed under royal patronage, and clear records were kept. All the major *sutras*, *tantras* and *shastras*[1] were translated from Sanskrit into Tibetan at that time, and the principal Indian Buddhist systems of practice were established as living traditions in the Land of Snows. Tibetans remember this as the golden era of the Three Great Dharma Kings.[2] Even though the civil wars of the early ninth century destroyed much of what had been accomplished, nonetheless many translations survived, as well as dictionaries of technical terms, and before long many of the lineages were revived. The schools of Tibetan Buddhism deriving from transmissions of this period are known as the Nyingmapa,[3] or "Old Schools." This term is synonymous with the phrase "the Early Dissemination of the Doctrine."

In the eleventh century increasing numbers of Tibetans once more began to travel south over the Himalayas to study with Indian masters. Many of them joined the training programs at the large international monastic universities of northern India, such as Nalanda and Vikramashila. Others studied with individual masters, as was the case in Marpa's training under Naropa. A movement to re-translate large sections of the vast corpus of Buddhist Sanskrit literature began, using a revised terminology based on Tibet's centuries-old Buddhist experience and on the nature of Buddhism in India at that time. The scholar-yogis returning to Tibet found themselves eagerly sought after as teachers; clusters of students grew up around them, and these developed into monasteries and hermitages dedicated to the study and practice of the specific lineages imported by the founding translator.

Because this Later Dissemination of the Doctrine was largely a freelance undertaking, in contrast to the Early Dissemination, which had generous court funding, the results were predictably individualistic. Several dozen new schools of Tibetan Buddhism were born at this time, the similarity between them being established by the fact that the language they used in their translations was somewhat standard, having followed the movement emanating from western Tibet.

Thus prior to Tsongkhapa's time most schools of Tibetan Buddhism were primarily based upon specific transmissions coming directly from India. The school that was to emanate from his work, known as the Gelukpa, or "Order of Excellence," was the only successful Tibetan Buddhist school to be formulated solely from a fusion of indigenous Tibetan lineages. Similar movements gradually became absorbed into the other schools, and thus ceased to exist as independent entities.

It didn't take Tsongkhapa long to discover that some lineages of transmission were more powerful than others, and that some had remained more true to the letter and spirit of Indian Buddhism. Even with the transmissions of the early masters whom he greatly admired, his impression was that, with the passage of the generations, many of the Tibetan lineage lamas had become somewhat provincial, and suffered from poor training, sloppy understanding, and spiritual complacency.

He made it his life's work to trace down the clearest of the many lineages of transmission coming from India, his measuring stick always having three edges to it: the original sutras and tantras spoken by the Buddha; the treatises (Skt. *shastras*) of the Indian masters; and the works of the early Tibetan translators who imported the individual traditions.

One of the early translators in whom he placed great faith was Marpa Lotsawa[4] (b. 1012), the forefather of the Kargyupa school (Tib. *bKa' brgyud ring lugs*; lit. "Order of Instructions"). Prominent among the lineages that Marpa imported was that famed as "Naro's Six Dharmas," i.e., the Six Yogas of Naropa.

Tsongkhapa's treatise on this system of tantric practice is formally entitled *A Book of Three Inspirations: A Treatise on the Stages of Training in the Profound Path of Naro's Six Dharmas* (hereafter simply referred to as *A Book of Three Inspirations*). It became the standard guide to the Naropa tradition at Ganden Monastery, the seat he founded near Lhasa in 1409. Ganden was to become the motherhouse of the Gelukpa school, and thus the symbolic head of the network of thousands of Gelukpa monasteries that sprang up over the succeeding centuries across Central Asia, from Siberia to northern India. *A Book of Three Inspirations* has served as the fundamental guide to Naropa's Six Yogas for the tens of thousands of Gelukpa monks, nuns and lay practitioners throughout that vast area who were interested in pursuing the Naropa tradition as a personal tantric study. It has performed that function for almost six centuries now.

Tsongkhapa's *Collected Works* contains two texts on the Six Yogas: *A Book of Three Inspirations*, which was actually composed by him, and is sixty folios or 120 pages in length; and an abbreviation and recasting of this work, compiled and edited by one of his disciples,

Sempa Chenpo Kunzangpa, which focuses on the actual meditations, leaving out the discussions of the principles involved. The latter is twenty folios or forty pages in length, a third the size of Tsongkhapa's original.

In the Fire Monkey Year (1836) Jey Sherab Gyatso, a monk-scholar who attained to prominence in the mid-nineteenth century, delivered a public reading of Lama Tsongkhapa's *A Book of Three Inspirations*. A disciple transcribed some of Jey Sherab Gyatso's words, and after the master's death these were published in his collected works under the title *Notes on A Book of Three Inspirations* (Tib. *Yid ches gsum ldan gyi bshad lung zin bris*). The opening passages of his text reveal something of the history of the tradition of Naropa's Six Yogas, and the attitude toward it in the Gelukpa school:

> Marpa of Lodrak received numerous transmissions directly from the illustrious (Indian) pandit Naropa. Among these were six instructions drawn from the various tantric traditions. He gathered these six into the structure that has become famed as "Naro's Six Dharmas." Each of these six contains a comprehensive presentation of the completion stage yogas; and the six as presented here provide a comprehensive approach to the completion stage yogas.
>
> Naropa imparted the Six Yogas to Marpa, together with the *Song of the Six Yogas*. However, even though all six of these certainly existed in India prior to Naropa, whether or not they had at that time been arranged into that structure is a point of doubt.
>
> Naropa's Six Yogas was the unique instruction of the early Kargyupa lamas. Lama Tsongkhapa the Great received this tradition and later composed his treatise on the system, *A Book of Three Inspirations*. Thus the Six Yogas came into the Gandenpa [i.e., Gelukpa] order.
>
> The Kargyupas are especially renowned for their tradition of the Six Yogas, and their early lineage masters, such as Marpa, Milarepa, Gampopa, Pakmo Drupa and Drikungpa, were flawless elucidators of the tradition. However, as the lineage passed from generation to generation a large number of subtle points of confusion and error found their way into many of the oral transmissions. Jey Gyalwa Nyipa [the "Second Buddha," i.e., Tsongkhapa] removed these, and clarified all the key points and basic principles of the system. For this reason the lineage of Naropa's Six Yogas as practiced within the Gelukpa order today is especially powerful.

The names given in the above passage identify the lineage of transmission of "Naro's Six Dharmas": Naropa himself (b. 1016), who was the Indian Buddhist master to train Marpa Lotsawa of Tibet in the doctrines and practices of the Six Yogas; Marpa Lotsawa (b. 1012), who brought the lineage to Tibet and taught it to hundreds of disciples there; Milarepa (b. 1040), one of Tibet's greatest poets, and also one of Marpa's four greatest disciples; Gampopa (b. 1079), the Doctor of Dakpo, a Kadampa monk who became a disciple of Milarepa and eventually emerged as the latter's most successful Dharma heir; glorious Pakmo Drupa (b. 1110), who was to inspire the vast popularity that Naropa's Six Yogas achieved in the twelfth century; and Drikungpa Jigten Sumgon (b. 1143), the most illustrious of Pakmo Drupa's eight chief disciples.

Thus here we have the names of Naropa and the first five generations of Tibetan lineage masters descending from him, beginning with Marpa Lotsawa. The schools originating in these lamas, known as the Kargyupa, were the early vehicle of Naropa's Six Yogas in Tibet.

Marpa had four chief disciples, all of whom received a number of unique lineages. Three of these—Ngokton, Tsurton and Milarepa—received the transmission of Naropa's Six Yogas. The fourth—Meytson—received Marpa's Guhyasamaja lineages. Tsongkhapa quotes or refers to all four extensively throughout his treatise, yet it was Milarepa's lineage of Naropa's Six Yogas that was to be received by Lama Tsongkhapa some three centuries later.

Milarepa in turn produced dozens of accomplished disciples in the traditions of the Six Yogas. The most charismatic of these was the Kadampa monk Gampopa, whose hermitage in Dakpo became a hive of activity, with yogis and yoginis immersing themselves in training under him. Four of these became predominant, and from these there came four separate Kargyupa sub-sects, known as the "four older Kargyupa schools" (Tib. *bKa' brgyud ring lugs che bzhi*). The glorious Pakmo Drupa, mentioned in the quotation above, was one of these four. He in turn produced eight most excellent disciples, from each of whom was born yet another separate Kargyupa sub-sect, known as the "eight younger Kargyupa schools" (Tib. *bKa' brgyud ring lugs chung brgyad*).[5] Thus there came to be twelve distinct Kargyupa sects, each holding individual transmissions of the Six Yogas. These generally had a central monastery or hermitage, and dozens of affiliated ones.

Tsongkhapa summarizes the list of the early Kargyupa lamas as follows in *A Book of Three Inspirations*:

> Marpa transmitted his lineage [of the Six Yogas of Naropa] to three of his disciples: Ngokton, Tsurton and Milarepa. In turn, Milarepa transmitted his lineages to two main disciples: Chojey Gampopa

and Rechungpa. The lineage descending from Gampopa multiplied into many different forms, each with its own specialty,
uniqueness and individual views on the different practices....

Thus within a hundred years of arriving in Tibet the tradition of
"Naro's Six Dharmas" had established a firm foothold in the Land of
Snows.

In the quotation above, Jey Sherab Gyatso begins by mentioning
these early Tibetan masters. He then jumps more than two centuries,
and introduces the author of our text, Tsongkhapa the Great, and the
role that he was to play in the transmission. The nineteenth-century
Jey Sherab Gyatso is, of course, a monk of the Gelukpa school descending from Lama Tsongkhapa. This is obvious from the words
with which he concludes his line of thought, "For this reason the lineage of Naropa's Six Yogas as practiced within the Gelukpa order
today is especially powerful." What he means is that Lama
Tsongkhapa applied the strength of his genius to the Six Yogas tradition, thus empowering the Gelukpa transmission with the unique
depth and lucidity that he brought into everything he touched, presenting each point within the context of the overall structure of Buddhist doctrine. Even a casual reading of his text reveals the richness
of his style, as he compares the diverse ideas floating around the Tibetan spiritual world at the time.

However, with Tsongkhapa the Great we are already into the late
fourteenth and early fifteenth centuries. Perhaps it would be useful
to jump back in time to the roots of tantric Buddhism in Tibet, which
lie in the Buddhist tantric tradition of ancient India.

THE BUDDHIST TANTRIC TRADITION IN INDIA

The Buddhist legacy of eleventh-century northern India, the period
in which Naropa and Marpa lived, was a blending of the *Sutrayana*,
or open, exoteric teachings of the Buddha (lit. "the Way of the Public
Discourses"), and the *Mantrayana*, or "Way of Secret Mantra," which
refers to the esoteric teachings of the tantric traditions. The Sutrayana
in turn is usually spoken of as having two facets: the *Hinayana*, or
"Streamlined Way Teachings," also sometimes called the *Shravakayana*,
or "Teachings Recorded by the Monk Disciples"; and the *Mahayana*,
or "Great Way," whose teachings were mostly given to saint-status
disciples (i.e., bodhisattvas). This latter is also referred to in traditional Buddhist literature as the *Bodhisattvayana*, or "Way of the

Universalist Warriors," and as the *Paramitayana,* or "Way of the Perfections." In traditional literature the Mantrayana is also referred to
by several other names, the two most common being the *Vajrayana,*
or "Diamond Way," and *Tantrayana,* or "Way of the Tantras." We will
see several references to these terms throughout Lama Tsongkhapa's
commentary as he discusses the various yogic techniques, meditations and philosophical attitudes embodied in the legacy of the Six
Yogas of Naropa.

Even though it is said that the tantras were taught by the Buddha
2,500 years ago, it seems that historically they began to emerge publicly in India in about the fourth or fifth centuries C.E. According to
tantric tradition, prior to this they had been transmitted in secret from
generation to generation.

Each tantra had a scripture that represented the quintessence of its
teaching (usually known as its *mulatantra,* or "root tantra"). It also
had a mandala of deities that symbolized it as a philosophy of being,
a path to enlightenment, and the resultant state of buddhahood (Tib.
gzhi lam 'bras bu, or "basis, path and fruit"). As a path, each tantric
system contained an infrastructure of meditational techniques and
yogic methods to be engaged by tantric trainees in their *sadhana,* or
daily practice routine.

Hundreds of different Buddhist tantric systems had surfaced in
India by the ninth century. The Indian masters later categorized these
into four basic types, known as *kriya, charya, yoga* and *maha-anuttara-
yoga,* or "purification," "action," "yoga," and "great highest yoga"
tantras. Every tantric system became associated with one or another
of these four. The six doctrines that comprise Naropa's Six Yogas are
all drawn from the fourth category, the maha-anuttara-yoga tantras.

Although there are considerable differences between the individual
tantric systems, they are similar in that they all arrange their vast
array of practices into what is known in Tibetan as *rimpa nyigyi naljor*
(Tib. *rim pa gnyis kyi rnal 'byor*), or "two stages of yogic application."
In the first three types of tantric systems these two are known as "the
yoga of symbols" and "the yoga beyond symbols." In maha-anuttara-
yoga tantra, they are called the "generation stage yogas" and the
"completion stage yogas." In this fourth category of tantras, the first
stage of practice mainly consists of visualizing oneself and all others
as mandala deities, cultivating an awareness of the world as a
mandala, generating the tantric pride, reciting the appropriate mantras, and so forth. The second stage of practice consists of physical

yogas and meditations on subtle physiology, such as those taught in the Six Yogas of Naropa and discussed in depth in Tsongkhapa's *A Book of Three Inspirations.*

The maha-anuttara-yoga tantras, or highest yoga tantra systems that flourished in north and northwest India during Naropa's lifetime, are those from which Naropa's Six Yogas are drawn: Guhyasamaja, Heruka Chakrasamvara, Hevajra, Yamantaka, Mahamaya, Shri Chaturpitha, and so forth.

In the early days of tantric Buddhism in India most tantras probably were practiced as individual, self-contained units. Each represented a complete *sadhana,* or path to enlightenment, and was adopted as such by tantric practitioners. By the ninth and tenth centuries, however, the tradition of practicing the various tantric lineages as separate systems had begun to fade.

The new trend was in what the Tibetans call *men ngak* (Tib. *man ngag*), or "oral tradition instructions." At first these were systems of practice that were formulated from quintessential elements within a given tantra; that is to say, they were simplifications of a more complex tantric system. But before long an alternative trend began to emerge, one in which elements from different tantric systems were being combined for maximum efficacy. The *men ngak* of this nature usually drew into one package many diverse yogic and philosophical ideas prevalent in the tantric world of Buddhist India during the time of their formulation. They are usually known by the name of either their formulator or promulgator, and are based on the state of enlightenment that he or she achieved by means of them. Examples would be "the Six Yogas" of the female mystic Sukhasiddhi; the longevity and healing yogas of the female tantric saint Siddharani; and, of course, the famous Six Yogas of Naropa, the subject of *A Book of Three Inspirations.*

NAROPA

Naropa was one of the preeminent Indian Buddhist masters of his time. He is particularly important in the history of Tibetan Buddhism, for his lineages became widespread throughout Tibet within a century of his demise. He played a dominant role in the dissemination of numerous tantras, most notably the Kalachakra,[6] Guhyasamaja, Hevajra and Chakrasamvara traditions, as well as in the promulgation of the fusion approach to the highest yoga tantras, exemplified by the Six Yogas transmission.

Naropa's biography has been related in several Western sources. The most authoritative and enchanting treatment is H. V. Guenther's *The Life and Teachings of Naropa* (Oxford University Press, 1963).[7] Prof. Guenther, one of the first Westerners to translate Tibetan into English with any degree of seriousness, here delivers a wonderful rendition of a fifteenth-century Tibetan account of Naropa's life, with a magically fabulous telling of Naropa's adventures during his twelve-year training under Tilopa.[8]

In Tibetan literature Naropa is usually referred to as a "drupchen" (Tib. *grub chen*; Skt. *mahasiddha*), a "great adept." Here the Sanskrit *maha* means great, and *siddha* indicates a person who has attained *siddhi*, or tantric accomplishment. These siddhis, or tantric accomplishments, are of two types: common, such as clairvoyance, being able to walk through walls, etc.; and exclusive, referring to the attainment of supreme enlightenment.

The mahasiddhas are always depicted as very eccentric, non-conventional characters, and generally are described as possessing great spiritual powers and magical abilities. Tibetan religious histories list the names of hundreds of Indian mahasiddhas who emerged during India's Vajrayana period. Eighty-four of them are special favorites of the Tibetans, and are often depicted in watercolor paintings as a set. Naropa is included among them. Tsongkhapa quotes both the original tantras and the treatises by the mahasiddhas extensively throughout his text.

Every Tibetan knows many stories from the life of Naropa by heart. Like Buddha, he had been born of an aristocratic family, but from childhood longed for the spiritual life. Like Buddha, he was forced into an arranged marriage; and, like Buddha, he later renounced it, together with his worldly position, to become a monk. Like Buddha, he endured great trials and hardships in the course of his training. And, like Buddha, he achieved perfect enlightenment.

Born in Bengal to a Buddhist family, in the early part of his life Naropa studied with numerous celebrated teachers, firstly in Bengal and then in Kashmir, where he was sent for his higher education. He achieved considerable renown for his efforts, eventually even becoming the abbot of Nalanda, India's most prestigious monastic university. He retained the abbotship for some eight years, achieving widespread fame as one of India's foremost Buddhist scholars.

However, during his fortieth year he experienced an encounter that radically affected the course of his life. At the time he was sitting quietly, reading a scripture. Suddenly he noticed an ugly old woman observing him. She inquired, "Do you understand the words of what you are reading?" Naropa replied in the affirmative. The old hag laughed and added, "And do you understand the essence?" Again Naropa replied in the affirmative, whereupon the old woman burst out in tears. "Here you are lying," she scolded.

Over the days and weeks to follow, the impact of the conversation played havoc on Naropa's mind, and eventually he came to the conclusion that he would have to leave Nalanda in search of a guru. Thus, shortly thereafter he resigned his seat in the monastery and left in search of a tantric master. After much wandering and many great trials, he encountered Tilopa.

Naropa's search for and then training under Tilopa is told in wildly mystical language, at once both allegorical and magical. He meets a leper woman and passes hastily by her; she sings him a verse on how, without compassion as one's motive and wisdom one's perspective, one can never find the guru.

Among his other encounters during his search were a man catching and eating lice, a man disemboweling a corpse, and so on. Each offers him a new clue on the spiritual attitude to be cultivated in order to become worthy to meet with the tantric guru.

Eventually Tilopa manifests to him, and an intense twelve-year training follows. Tibetans love to tell and re-tell how, under Tilopa, Naropa dedicated himself to the training; how Tilopa pushed him to the limits of human endurance, and yet he persisted; and how eventually he achieved full enlightenment and became a mahasiddha.

In the later part of his life Naropa attracted many disciples from India, Nepal, Tibet and the other Buddhist regions to the north of the sub-continent. However, historically speaking his most successful transmissions were those that he gave to Marpa Lotsawa, for these came to grow and multiply, eventually penetrating the structure of almost all Central Asian Buddhist sects.

The lineages brought to Tibet by Marpa Lotsawa and transmitted by the early Kargyupa lamas became a major pillar in the spiritual mansion being constructed by Tsongkhapa the Great. He especially cherished the Naropa transmissions, as indicated by the tone of *A Book of Three Inspirations*. The text was to establish a prominent place for "Naro's Six Dharmas" within the rapidly blossoming Gelukpa school.

THE LEGACY OF THE SIX YOGAS

Generally it is said that the formulator of the Six Yogas of Naropa in fact was not Naropa himself, as the name would suggest, but rather his guru Tilopa (b. 988). Yet, as Jey Sherab Gyatso (b. 1803) states in the pasasge quoted above, "even though all six of these certainly existed in India prior to Naropa, whether or not they had at that time been arranged into that structure is a point of doubt." Although Tilopa and Naropa had brought together numerous elements from diverse tantric sources, and Naropa had transmitted these to Marpa Lotsawa, it is a point of doubt precisely who had given the system the sixfold structure by which it became known in Tibet.

Moreover, Tsongkhapa suggests in his discussion of the elements comprising the six individual yogas that even though "Naro's Six Dharmas" represent the essence of the transmissions given by Naropa to Marpa, it is probable that Marpa also drew from at least four of his numerous Nepalese and Indian gurus—Chiterpa, who was Nepalese, and Naropa, Jnanagarbha and Maitripa, who were Indians—in formulating the structure and presentation of the transmission to become famed as "Naro's Six Dharmas." Naropa was Marpa's main guru, but the other three played major roles in his spiritual training.

Tsongkhapa also points out that there are various ways of counting and structuring the six. In settling upon the arrangement that he prefers, he refers to the writings of glorious Pakmo Drupa (b. 1110), one of the early lineage masters, wherein the structure is as follows: (1) inner heat; (2) illusory body; (3) clear light; (4) consciousness transference; (5) forceful projection; and (6) the bardo yoga.

The tradition of speaking of this legacy from Marpa Lotsawa as being sixfold seems to have evolved somewhat randomly. As Tsongkhapa puts it,"There are many ways of structuring this system of tantric yogas, the most common being into two, three, four, six and ten branches." In other words, the system could just as easily have ended up being popularly known as "Naro's Two Dharmas," "Naro's Four Dharmas," "Naro's Ten Dharmas," and so forth, without omitting any actual substance from the transmission

The twofold manner of structuring the Six Yogas of Naropa is given in a treatise by Gyalwa Wensapa (b. 1505), a Gelukpa yogi who spent over twenty years meditating in caves and hermitages, achieving enlightenment in one lifetime. He was also an early lineage holder of the Six Yogas transmission, and his name appears in the Seventh Dalai

Lama's lineage prayer (translated below). His text, entitled *A Source of Every Realization: The Stamp of the Six Yogas of Naropa* (Tib. *Na ro chos drug gi lag rjes dngos grub kun 'byung*), speaks of (1) the yogas for drawing the vital energies into the central channel; and (2) the yogas that are performed once the energies have been withdrawn in this way. Here the inner heat yoga represents the first of these, and the remaining five yogas are subsumed under the second outline.

The Six Yogas are spoken of as three when they are arranged as follows: (1) the foundation, which is comprised of the inner heat yoga; (2) the main body of the practice, which includes the illusory body and clear light yogas; and (3) the auxiliary trainings, which include the yogas of consciousness transference and forceful projection. Here the bardo yoga is subsumed under the illusory body yoga. This is mentioned by Tsongkhapa.

Marpa Lotsawa seems mainly to have spoken of them as fourfold: (1) inner heat; (2) *karmamudra*, or sex yogas; (3) illusory body; and (4) clear light. Here three of the six—i.e., those of consciousness transference, forceful projection and the bardo yogas—are not given the status of separate "Dharmas," presumably because they are relegated to the position of auxiliary practices.

Tsongkhapa quotes the yogi Milarepa as using a somewhat different sixfold classification:

> The tradition of Marpa of the Southern Hills has six instructions: (1) the generation stage yogas; (2) inner heat; (3) karmamudra yogas; (4) introduction to the essence of the view of the ultimate nature of being; (5) the indicative clear light of the path; and (6) the indicative illusory nature, together with dream yoga. This is the heart-essence of Marpa's teachings. There is no higher precept for introducing the trainee to the essence of the whispered teachings. There is no more precious instruction than this, the heart of that yogi's thought. No teaching is more practical.

Although Tsongkhapa mentions a tenfold structure for the system, he does not list the ten. This arrangement may be found, however, in a commentary by Ngulchu Dharmabhadra entitled *An Ornament for A Book of Three Inspirations* (Tib. *Na ro chos drug gi zin bris yid ches dgongs rgyan*). Ngulchu states,

> Then there is a tenfold manner of structuring the system: (1) the generation stage yogas; (2) the view of emptiness; (3) the inner heat; (4) karmamudra yogas; (5) the illusory body; (6) the clear

light; (7) dream yoga; (8) the bardo yogas; (9) consciousness transference; and (10) forceful projection.

If we compare this list of ten to the six as given by Pakmo Drupa and Tsongkhapa, we will see that all ten have been incorporated within the six.

Ngulchu also lists the manner in which Pakmo Drupa presents the Six Yogas, which is the structure followed by Tsongkhapa in *A Book of Three Inspirations*, and then gives an alternative formulation. This is an interesting variation, and Ngulchu introduces it in order to show how Tsongkhapa chose the title of his text. As he puts it,

> Tsongkhapa also spoke of another sixfold structure: (1) inner heat and (2) karmamudra yogas, which are derived from the Hevajra Tantra; (3) illusory body and (4) clear light, which are derived from the Guhyasamaja Tantra; and, finally, (5) consciousness transference and (6) forceful projection, which emanate from the Shri Chaturpitha Tantra.... Because these three sets of two are derived from such authoritative sources, Tsongkhapa entitles his text *A Book of Three Inspirations*.

These three Indian tantric systems are referred to repeatedly throughout Tsongkhapa's text, for they are essential sources of the Six Yogas. Note that here the bardo doctrine is not mentioned separately, as it is included under the illusory body yoga; in its place, karmamudra yoga is elevated to the status of one of the six yogas.

As Ngulchu Dharmabhadra states above, and as Tsongkhapa points out several times in his treatise, Naropa's Six Yogas were comprised of elements drawn from the principal tantras popular in northern India at the time. This is stated as follows in the concluding verses of *A Book of Three Inspirations*,

> The incomparable Buddha Shakyamuni, lord of sages,
> Taught the holy Dharma for the benefit of living beings.
> Supreme of his teachings are those of highest yoga tantra,
> Both the female tantras and the male tantras.

> From the female tantras [i.e., Hevajra and Chakrasamvara]
> Comes the teaching on the inner heat doctrine, *chandali*,
> A method for bringing the subtle energies under control
> And arousing the innate wisdom.

> With this as the basis one takes up the practice
> Of the illusory body and clear light doctrines
> That emanate from the Guhyasamaja Tantra,

And the doctrines of consciousness transference
And forceful projection to another residence
That emanate from the Shri Chaturpitha Tantra.

Based on those sources there arose
This tradition from the mahasiddhas Tilopa and Naropa
Famed as "the Six Yogas of Naropa."
Countless practitioners here in this land of snows
Have delighted in this festival of profound tantric endeavor,
A deeply cherished and precious oral tradition legacy.

In another section of his treatise Lama Tsongkhapa speaks of the various sources of the Six Yogas. For example, he suggests that Marpa Lotsawa drew some of the material in the doctrines of the illusory body and clear light from another of his Indian gurus, Jnanagarbha, with whom Marpa had studied the Guhyasamaja Tantra. Guhyasamaja is the source from which Naropa's Six Yogas take the illusory body and clear light doctrines. Tsongkhapa states,

> The instruction on the inner heat yoga comes to us through Tilopa, who commented that this was the transmission of the mahasiddha Krishnacharya, also known [to Tibetans] as Lobpon Acharyapa. Here these previously existent oral traditions are used as the basis. This is enriched and clarified in reference to *The Sambhuta Drop of Springtime* (Skt. *Samputa tilaka*) and also Acharya Krishnacharya's *The Drop of Springtime* (Skt. *Vasanta tilaka*).
>
> The illusory body and the clear light doctrines are derived from the Guhyasamaja oral tradition, as taught by the Indian mahasiddha Jnanagarbha and received [by Marpa directly from him]. Thus these are based on the Guhyasamaja Tantra. Here the Marpa tradition of the Guhyasamaja oral instruction transmission has been used as the basis, with references to the Guhyasamaja cycle of the Aryas, Father and Sons [i.e., "The Arya Cycle of Guhyasamaja Doctrines"].
>
> The practices of consciousness transference and forceful projection to a new residence are based on the Four Seats Tantra (Skt. *Shri chaturpitha tantra*). In addition,...they are associated with numerous other tantric traditions, including the Sambhuta Tantra, the Vajradaka Tantra, and so forth.

The legacy of the Six Yogas thus appears to have roots in diverse Indian Buddhist tantric sources.

Another lineage of the Six Yogas known as the Six Yogas of Niguma was transmitted to Tibet through Niguma, a female disciple of Naropa who also received from him a transmission of the Six Yogas. This alternative lineage was not brought to Tibet by Marpa Lotsawa, but rather by one of his contemporaries, a lama by the name of Kyungpo Naljor.[9] The main difference between the two transmissions seems to be that the Niguma system replaces the yoga of forceful projection with dream yoga.

Jey Sherab Gyatso (b. 1803) makes a statement to this effect in his *Notes on A Book of Three Inspirations* (Tib. *Yid ches gsum ldan gyi bshad lung zin bris*),

> Originally the dream yogas were not emphasized in the system of the Six Yogas of Naropa; and the yoga of forceful projection did not exist in the system of the Six Yogas of Niguma. It seems that this difference is the reason for maintaining these two as separate systems. Otherwise, the two are very similar.

In *Notes on A Book of Three Inspirations* Jey Sherab Gyatso also points out that

> Each of these six [yogas] contains a comprehensive presentation of the completion stage yogas; and the six as presented here provide a comprehensive approach to the completion stage yogas.

The implication is that the system can be taken as an integrated and holistic approach to the completion stage yogas, in which case all six practiced together as a unit represent the essence of all completion stage practices; alternatively, any one of the six can be taken as the principal focus of one's practice, in which case all completion stage yogas are approached from and drawn into it. These days the former tradition is more common, although the biographies of yogis of bygone centuries suggest that this was not always the case.

Gyalwa Wensapa sums up the situation as follows in *A Source of Every Realization: The Stamp of the Six Yogas of Naropa* (Tib. *Na ro chos drug gi lag rjes dngos grub kun 'byung*),

> Thus the jewel-like practitioner who engages in the profound path of Naropa's Six Yogas has entered into a complete and unmistaken path for accomplishing enlightenment in one short lifetime, even in this degenerate age.

THE SIX YOGAS, THREE BARDO STATES, AND NINE BLENDINGS

Lama Tsongkhapa states in the opening section of *A Book of Three Inspirations* that

> It is recorded that when Venerable Milarepa taught the oral instruction transmission for achieving liberation in the bardo he

said, "First establish the basics...." The above expression, "the oral instruction transmission for achieving liberation in the bardo," is synonymous [with the Six Yogas of Naropa].

In other words, in the time of Milarepa (b. 1040) the Six Yogas of Naropa were also known by the name "the Bardo Trang-dol system" (Tib. *bar do 'phrang sgrol*), which translates as "the Oral Transmission for Achieving Liberation in the Bardo."

Most readers will be familiar with the Tibetan term "bardo," which literally means "the in-between," and its reference to the after-death state. Several translations of the *Bardo To-dol* (Tib. *Bar do thos sgrol*), or "Liberation by Hearing in the Bardo," have appeared in English under the title *The Tibetan Book of the Dead*, resulting in "bardo" being the first (and perhaps only) Tibetan word to find its way into the Oxford and Webster's dictionaries.

A unique feature of the Six Yogas tradition is that it speaks of three bardo states, and of the methods of practicing tantric meditation in each of them. The three are: the bardo of the waking state between birth and death; the bardo of sleep and dreams; and the bardo between death and rebirth. Only the third of the three usages of the term *bardo* carries the sense that it has in *The Tibetan Book of the Dead*.

The Six Yogas tradition speaks of how the tantric technology is to be applied in each of these three bardo states. This process is known as "the yoga of the three blendings in the three situations." In other words, the three blendings are to be engaged in each of the three bardo states, and thus there are nine "blendings." Because by means of the Six Yogas one can practice in all three bardo states—waking, sleeping/dreaming, and after death—the tradition was called "the Oral Transmission for Achieving Liberation in the Bardo."

To understand what is being referred to by the "nine blendings," we must have a basic knowledge of the Mahayana Buddhist concept of the three *kayas*: *Dharmakaya, Sambhogakaya,* and *Nirmanakaya.*

The doctrine of the three kayas is fundamental to all highest yoga tantra systems. Volumes have been written on the subject in the Tibetan language. The idea is that at the time of enlightenment the mind of the practitioner transforms into the Dharmakaya, speech transforms into the Sambhogakaya, and the body manifests as the Nirmanakaya. The Dharmakaya can only be perceived by other buddhas; the Sambhogakaya can be perceived by aryas, or highly realized beings; and the Nirmanakaya can be perceived by ordinary beings. Therefore it is said that the Dharmakaya fulfills one's own wishes and needs, whereas the Sambhogakaya and Nirmanakaya fulfill the wishes and needs of the world. Sometimes the Sambhogakaya and Nirmanakaya are grouped together as the Rupakaya, or "Form Body," in which case only two kayas are mentioned: Dharmakaya, which fulfills one's own purposes; and Rupakaya, which fulfills the purposes of others.

In exoteric Mahayana practice the emphasis is on cultivating the mind, the speech or communicative principle, and the body, until they eventually grow into these three kayas. In tantric Buddhism, something from the enlightenment state of the three kayas is brought into and blended with our ordinary situation. For this reason the exoteric Mahayana is sometimes called "the causal vehicle," i.e., the path in which one meditates upon the causes of enlightenment and thus grows into it; and the esoteric tantric path "the resultant vehicle," because in it one brings something from the resultant state of enlightenment into ordinary experience. In other words, the idea behind the "three blendings" is that on certain occasions we can take an element from within the body-mind complex and its stream of experience, and use this as a proxy (Tib. *rjes mthun*) of one of the three kayas, or enlightenment dimensions, supplementing the natural force of this proxy with the forces of meditation and yogic application.

The concept of blending with the three kayas is first introduced during the generation stage practice, in which one meditates upon oneself as a tantric deity dwelling at the center of the supporting mandala. Here one engages in the process known as "taking the three kayas as the path" (Tib. *sku gsum lam 'khyer*), which refers to three steps in meditation: (1) the visualization that the world and its inhabitants dissolve into one's body, and then the coarse energies withdraw from within one's body, just as at the time of death, until the clear light mind arises, which is known as "taking death as the Dharmakaya"; (2) the visualization that one arises from the clear light in a pure energy form, which is the practice of taking the bardo experience as the Sambhogakaya; and (3) the visualization that one arises as the Mandala Lord, which is the process of taking rebirth as the Nirmanakaya. This generation stage meditation is performed daily by all serious initiates, and in the Six Yogas system sets the stage for the completion stage trainings of the "three blendings."

As Tsongkhapa explains, in the completion stage yogas this principle is extended to three different environments: blending with the three kayas during the waking state; blending with the three kayas during sleep; and blending with the three kayas at the time of death. In other words, the three blendings are performed in each of the three bardo states. The underlying concept here is that the life process itself is a metaphor for the three kayas, and we can utilize this parallel in our yogic application during each of the three bardo states.

It may be useful to look at some of the ways in which the Six Yogas are presented by the different Tibetan commentators in order to appreciate what is being said here.

Tsongkhapa states in *A Book of Three Inspirations* that the Six Yogas actually could be presented as three: (1) the foundation of the path, which is the inner heat yoga; (2) the main body of the path, which includes both the illusory body and clear light doctrines; and (3) the auxiliary trainings, which are comprised of the consciousness transference and forceful projection doctrines. When we compare this to how Gyalwa Wensapa condenses the Six Yogas, based on their function, into two, we can see something of what the "blendings" are about. The two are: (1) those yogas for drawing the vital energies into the central channel; and (2) those that are applied after the energies have been drawn into the central channel. Here Tsongkhapa's first category, the inner heat yoga, is also Gyalwa Wensapa's first. Tsongkhapa's remaining two, and Wensapa's second, contain the remaining five yogas of the Six Yogas system.

Why, in the context of the "three blendings," is the inner heat yoga called "the foundation state," and the illusory body and clear light yogas called "the actual path"? Because by means of the inner heat yoga one gains control over the coarse and subtle energies of the body; these energies are withdrawn, causing the according inner and outer signs to manifest, together with the related visions, until the clear light of mind arises just as at the time of death. In other words, it is by means of the inner heat yoga that the clear light consciousness can be invoked in the continuum of one's conscious experience. This is blended with a proxy of the Dharmakaya. The illusory body technology is then applied in order to blend with the Sambhogakaya and Nirmanakaya. Thus the inner heat is the foundation of the three blendings, but the clear light and illusory body yogas are the actual method of engaging the blendings.

One of the most wonderfully succinct presentations of this process of the three blendings is that found in the treatise by Gyalwa Wensapa, *A Source of Every Realization: The Stamp of the Six Yogas of Naropa*:

The technology for drawing the vital energies into the central channel begins with generating the image of oneself as Buddha Vajradhara, male and female in sexual union, and envisioning the energy channels, together with the mantric syllables at the chakras, meditating on the heat, and finally meditating on the melting drops. This causes the vital energies to enter, abide and dissolve.

The sign indicating the entering of the vital energies is that, when a breath is inhaled in order to test one's progress, the air flows evenly through both nostrils. The sign indicating that they have been caused to abide is that the visions of the elemental dissolutions and also the dissolution of the three visionary states occur. These dissolutions must be individually recognized. Earth dissolves into water, and there is a vision like seeing a mirage; water dissolves into fire, and there is a smoke-like vision; fire dissolves into air, and there is a vision like flickering fireflies. Then the air element begins to dissolve into the visionary consciousness called "appearance." There is a vision like that of the glow of a butterlamp. Air fully dissolves into "appearance," and there is a vision of whiteness, like a clear autumn sky pervaded by the light of the full moon. This dissolves into the consciousness known as "proximity," and there is a vision of redness, like that of the clear sky pervaded by sunlight. This dissolves into "proximate attainment," and there is a vision of overwhelming darkness, like the sky before dawn, with neither sun nor moon. "Proximate attainment" then dissolves into the clear light; there is a vision of clear radiance, like the sky at daybreak, free from the three conditions. One must recognize these experiences as they occur. This is the process known as "blending with Dharmakaya during the waking state."

When the time comes to arise from the clear light absorption one arouses the strong instinct to put aside one's old aggregates and arise in the form of a Buddha Vajradhara, male and female in union. Then when one arises from the clear light one's old aggregates will be set aside and within the mind there forms the image of a Buddha Vajradhara, male and female in union. Simultaneously one applies the technology for inducing the stages of dissolution [described above] in reverse order. Thus one goes from the clear light to proximate attainment, to proximity, and to appearance. One experiences the signs of the elemental dissolutions [in reverse]: a glow like that of a butterlamp; firefly-like sparks; smoke; and finally the mirage. This is the process known as "blending with the Sambhogakaya during the waking state."

One engages in the stages of meditation on transformations associated with that Sambhogakaya form, and focuses one's absorption upon it. When one decides to arise from the absorption, one does so by meditating upon one's old aggregates as the Symbolic Being [Skt. *samayasattva*], with the Wisdom Being [Skt. *jnanasattva*] at the heart. This is the process known as "blending with Nirmanakaya during the waking state."

Simultaneous to this, as the air begins to flow through the nostrils again and the five sensory consciousnesses are revived, whatever appearances occur are seen as emptiness, emptiness as ecstasy, and ecstasy as the mandala and its deities. This is the practice to be cultivated in the post-meditation sessions.

Gyalwa Wensapa then explains the process of blending with the three kayas during the sleep and dream states,

Similarly, when that yogi goes to sleep he attempts to retain the clear light of sleep, and sets the resolution to arise as a Sambhogakaya deity in the dream state. As he prepares for sleep he engages in the meditations on the channels, energies and chakras, causing the drops to melt and the blisses to arise. The vital energies enter, abide and dissolve within the central channel. All the signs of the dissolution process occur, from "earth into water," until the emergence of the clear light. The four emptinesses emerge in the nature of the four blisses. At the same time as the clear light occurs, the yogi engages in meditation on ecstasy conjoined with [the wisdom of] emptiness. This is the process known as "blending with Dharmakaya in sleep."

When the time comes to arise from that clear light one generates the resolution to arise with a dream body by setting aside the body of the old aggregates and taking the form of a Buddha Vajradhara, male and female in union. Then when one emerges from the clear light [of sleep] the dream body appears, not as the body of the old aggregates, but rather as a Buddha Vajradhara, male and female in union. This is what is known as "blending with Sambhogakaya in dreams."

One focuses one's absorption on the meditations of the transformative processes of that Sambhogakaya. When the time comes to awaken from sleep, one does so by emerging with one's old aggregates envisioned as the Symbolic Being, and with the Wisdom Being at one's heart. This is the process known as "blending with Nirmanakaya while awakening."

Simultaneous to this, as the air begins to flow through the nostrils and the five sensory consciousnesses revive, whatever appearances occur are seen as emptiness, emptiness as ecstasy, and ecstasy as the mandala deities. This is the practice to be cultivated in the post-meditation sessions.

Thirdly Gyalwa Wensapa speaks of how the three blendings are engaged at the time of death and in the bardo,

The yogi who is not able to accomplish the realizations of the highest stage before the time of death should cultivate the resolution to apply the technology for retaining the clear light of death, arising in the Sambhogakaya in the bardo, and taking birth with the incarnation of a tantric master, a *mantracharyin*. Then as the actual moment of death draws near one should meditate on the channels, energies, chakras and so forth as above, and meditate upon the blazing and melting. This causes the vital energies to enter into the central channel, and to abide and dissolve, giving rise to the signs of the dissolutions, until the signs of the clear light occur. As the clear light of death emerges one focuses in meditation upon emptiness. This is the process known as "blending with Dharmakaya at death."

When the time comes to arise from the clear light one arouses the instinct to set aside the old aggregates and, in taking a bardo body, to arise in the form of a Buddha Vajradhara, male and female in union. Then as one emerges from the clear light the image of the bardo body arises, with the old aggregates set aside, and appearing as Buddha Vajradhara, male and female in union. Simultaneously the signs of the dissolution process manifest in reverse, as consciousness reverses through the stages of clear light to proximate attainment, and so forth, until the vision of the mirage. This is the process known as "blending with Sambhogakaya in the bardo."

One remains focused on the stages of absorption in the meditations of the Sambhogakaya transformations. Then when the wish to take rebirth begins to crystallize, one seeks a suitable genetic environment in the white and red drops [i.e., the fertilized egg] of one's future parents, in order to achieve rebirth as the special body-vessel of a mantracharyin. This is the process known as "blending with Nirmanakaya at rebirth."

Thus the ability to control the subtle energies and bring them into the central channel is indispensable to success in the process of the three blendings in the three situations. This control is established by the inner heat yoga, the foundation. As Tsongkhapa puts it, the inner heat located in the navel chakra is to be ignited, the energies brought into the central channel, and the subtle genetic drops melted. These "melted drops," which support the subtle energies of the body-mind complex, are then collected inside the heart chakra, where they are assembled as the basis of the subtle body. The energies from all other parts of the body are withdrawn into this unprecedented "house of the subtle mind," from which the clear light mind is to be consciously experienced for the first time.

Throughout *A Book of Three Inspirations* we see a constant repetition of the topic of the dissolution process, wherein the energies are withdrawn from each of the coarse elements. This begins with the earth energies dissolving into those of water; an inner vision is experienced, like that of a mirage. The water energies dissolve into fire, and the vision of smoke occurs. These stages of the energy dissolutions continue, until all the coarse energies have been withdrawn.

The subtle drops then come to the heart chakra. Firstly the red female drops collect, giving rise to a red vision and the mindset called "appearance." Secondly the white male drops collect; there is the inner vision of a white light, and one experiences the mindset known as "proximity." Thirdly the white and red drops collapse together; there is an inner vision of utter blackness, the mindset of "proximate attainment," and one swoons into unconsciousness. From this one arises in the fourth mindset, that of the primordial clear light. These four are also called the "four emptinesses."

The idea in highest yoga tantra is that we naturally experience these dissolutions in the three bardo states—our daily waking life, the sleep state, and the time of death. The "dissolution process," which is partially experienced every time we go to sleep, and is inescapably and utterly experienced at the time of death, can be consciously induced during the waking stage by means of tantric yoga. When we become skilled in inducing the dissolutions in our daily meditations, we become fluent in applying the same techniques during sleep and dreams, as well as at the time of death.

In Tsongkhapa's threefold breakdown of the system, the ability to consciously work with this dissolution process, and thus the ability to consciously induce the tantric blisses at will, is established by means of the inner heat yoga, which therefore is termed "the foundation stone." The main practice, the illusory body and clear light yogas, involves using the dissolution process firstly to manifest the illusory body, and then to immerse this illusory body in the clear light. One applies the technology of the dissolutions for producing the "unpurified" and "purified" illusory bodies, and realizing the "semblant" and "actual" clear light consciousnesses. This brings about enlightenment, which in the tantric tradition is known as *yuganaddha*, or "the great union." The auxiliary practices, i.e., the remaining three yogas, are merely aids in implementing the first three.

In *A Source of Every Realization: The Stamp of the Six Yogas of Naropa*, Gyalwa Wensapa explains the manner in which the practitioner is transported across the stages in training, until enlightenment is won:

> First one meditates on the phases of the dissolution process, which causes the vital energies to enter into the central channel, abide and dissolve. This gives rise to the signs of the dissolutions, from the mirage up to the clear light. When the time comes to emerge from the clear light, one arouses the resolution to have the unpurified illusory body transform into a purified illusory body. Then as one arises from the clear light the unpurified illusory body is set aside, and the image of the purified illusory body arises within the mind. Simultaneous to that, one experiences the dissolution process in reverse; one moves from the clear light to proximate attainment, and so forth, until the sign of the mirage. The being engaging that Sambhogakaya form then arises as Nirmanakaya, emanating forth the supported and supporting mandalas. When he wants to arise from meditation he does so by envisioning his old aggregates as the Symbolic Being, with the Wisdom Being at his heart....
>
> The practitioner of this illusory body stage cultivates these advanced meditations, and eventually sees signs that the accomplishment of the stage known as "the great union of training" is approaching. He engages in the practice of uniting with a karmamudra as the external condition; and as the inner condition engages the meditations on the stages of the dissolutions and so forth, causing the vital energies to enter the central channel, abide and dissolve. The signs of the dissolutions occur, from that of the mirage to that of the clear light. The four emptinesses emerge in the nature of the four blisses. At the moment of the innate clear light, one engages the meditation of ecstasy conjoined with emptiness.
>
> At that time five factors occur simultaneously: the state known as "proximate attainment in the unfoldment process" ceases; the innate ecstasy induces an unprecedented direct realization of emptiness; the illusory body is purified in the actual clear light and appears like a rainbow in a radiant sky; one achieves the unhindered stage wherein the direct antidote to the emotional obscurations is born within one's mindstream; and one's continuum becomes that of an arya.
>
> By the time the process of emerging from the clear light begins, one's previous driving force in the practice will have come into play, placing one at the door through which the "purified illusory body" can be achieved. As one emerges from the clear light, with

the role of the substantial cause being played by the subtle energy of five radiances, upon which rides the innate actuality [i.e., the innate actual clear light consciousness], and the role of the simultaneously present condition being played by the mind itself, one arises in the actual "purified illusory body," which flows in an unbroken stream in a form such as that of Buddha Vajradhara, male and female in union, adorned by the marks and signs of perfection, one's old aggregates set aside.

Simultaneously the signs of the dissolution process in reverse manifest, from that of going from the clear light to proximate attainment, until the sign of the mirage. At that time five factors occur: the innate actuality [i.e., actual clear light mind] ceases; the state of proximate attainment in the dissolution process is produced; the arisal of the "purified illusory body"; one achieves the path of utter liberation which is free from emotional obscurations; and one's continuum becomes that of an arhat. The being of that Sambhogakaya form then focuses in meditative absorption.

What are the stages of that absorption? One focuses in single-pointed meditation upon emptiness, and then causes the vital energies to enter into the central channel, to abide and to dissolve, giving rise to the signs, until the clear light occurs. At that time one has arrived at the place wherein can be unobstructedly achieved the state of great union, wherein body and mind can be assembled as a single entity. Here body is represented by the perfect illusory body adorned with the marks and signs of perfection; mind is represented by the actual clear light consciousness.

When the time comes to arise from that clear light one's previous driving force from the practice comes into play, and one finds oneself at the door through which the body of great union in training can become that of the great union beyond training. In emerging from the clear light, the being on the stage of "the great union of training" perceives the image of the body of the stage of "the great union beyond training." Simultaneously the signs of the reversal process occur, from that of moving from the clear light to proximate attainment, and so forth, until the mirage.

That Sambhogakaya holds the potential of the Nirmanakaya, which emanates forth a net of activities, such as manifesting the supported and supporting mandalas.

When one wishes to arise from meditation, one enters into one's own old aggregates or some other old aggregates, whichever is appropriate. Then, residing in that vessel, one shows Dharma to those to be trained, and cultivates the after-practice activities, such as uniting with a karmamudra, eating and drinking, as well as running with wild animals, and so forth....

The yogi on the stage of great union of training cultivates the absorptions of that level during both formal meditation and post-meditation sessions, and eventually sees signs of the approach of the attainment of great union beyond training. He engages the external condition of uniting with a karmamudra, and the internal condition of meditating single-pointedly on emptiness, causing the vital energies to enter into the central channel, and to abide and dissolve. The signs, beginning with the mirage and so forth, occur, until eventually the signs of the clear light manifest. The four emptinesses arise in the nature of the four blisses.

The moment this innate clear light manifests, one engages the meditation of ecstasy conjoined with [the wisdom of] emptiness. The first moment of this clear light is the unobstructed stage on which the perceptual obscurations are transcended. The second moment of it is also the first moment of omniscient buddhahood, wherein one remains in perfect absorption upon the final nature of being, while at the same time directly seeing all conventional realities as clearly as a piece of fruit held in the hand. The body of great union of training becomes the great union beyond training, the actual Sambhogakaya endowed with the kisses of the seven excellences, and that sends out thousands of Nirmanakaya emanations to benefit those to be trained. Thus one achieves complete buddhahood in the nature of the three kayas.

Thus we can see that the language of the "elemental dissolutions," "three blendings," and "three kayas" continues throughout the various levels of application of the Six Yogas of Naropa, which culminate in omniscient enlightenment, the state known as "the great union beyond training."

One of the most popular practice manuals on the Six Yogas system used by Gelukpa lamas today is *A Source of Great Ecstasy Realization: A Guide to the Profound Six Yogas of Naropa* (Tib. *Zab lam na ro'i chos drug gi khrid yig bde chen dngos grub 'byung nas*), by Nagtsang Tulku (mid-nineteenth century). Nagtsang divides the stages of practice into two: (1) meditating on the inner heat yoga in order to give rise to the four blisses; and (2) on the basis of that realization, the meditations on "the (nine) blendings." In other words, the practitioner is first instructed on how to apply the inner heat yoga in order to gain experience of the four blisses; these four are experienced by means of invoking the dissolution of the elemental energies, bringing the vital energies into the central channel, and melting the subtle drops. When this realization has been made firm, he or she is instructed in the technology of the "nine blendings" described above.

In summary, Gyalwa Wensapa's *A Source of Every Realization: The Stamp of the Six Yogas of Naropa* also looks at the process of the Six Yogas in reverse, i.e., from the stage of final enlightenment, or "great union beyond training," to the first step on the path:

> As a preliminary to attaining the stage of the great union beyond training, one must go through the stage of great union of training. As a preliminary to that one must accomplish the illusory body and clear light yogas, and to succeed in that one must first meditate upon the channels, chakras, blazing, melting, and so forth, as taught in the inner heat yoga.
>
> In turn, as a preliminary [to these completion stage practices] one must go to the end of the coarse and subtle generation stage practices in which one visualizes birth, death, and bardo, the bases to be purified, as the paths of the three kayas. For this one must have received the complete empowerments, and be mature in observing the disciplines adopted at the time of initiation. Moreover, before entering into tantric practice one should train the mind in the common path, from cultivating an effective working relationship with a spiritual master, up to the meditative training that combines shamata and vipasyana.
>
> Thus the jewel-like practitioner who engages in the profound path of Naropa's Six Yogas in this way has entered into a complete and unmistaken path for accomplishing enlightenment in one short lifetime, even in this degenerate age.

LAMA TSONGKHAPA'S *A BOOK OF THREE INSPIRATIONS*

The tradition of the Six Yogas became a major subject of Tibetan commentarial writing—treatises on the subject no doubt number well into the thousands. Over the centuries nearly every monastery produced one or more literary treatments of the system, perhaps mainly in order to provide a guide to how the Six Yogas could be integrated into the spiritual doctrines and linguistic infrastructure that formed the basis of its individual traditions. There were well over five thousand monasteries in the Tibetan ethnographic area prior to the great destructions wrought by the Communists earlier in this century. Many of these commentaries were lost in this destruction, but several hundred have survived and come down to us today.

Tsongkhapa the Great's *A Book of Three Inspirations* has for centuries been regarded as special among the many. The text occupies a unique place in Tibetan tantric literature, for it in turn came to serve as the basis of hundreds of later treatments. His observations on various dimensions and implications of the Six Yogas became a launching pad for hundreds of later yogic writers, opening up new horizons on the practice and philosophy of the system. In particular, his work is treasured for its panoramic view of the Six Yogas, discussing each of the topics in relation to the bigger picture of tantric Buddhism, tracing each of the yogic practices to its source in an original tantra spoken by the Buddha, and presenting each within the context of the whole.

His treatise is especially revered for the manner in which it discusses the first of the Six Yogas, that of the "inner heat." As His Holiness the present Dalai Lama put it at a public reading of and discourse upon the text in Dharamsala, India, in 1991, "the work is regarded by Tibetans as *tummo gyi gyalpo*, the king of treatments on the inner heat yoga." Few other Tibetan treatises match it in this respect.

Tsongkhapa wrote his commentary to the Six Yogas at the request of none other than the Pakmo Drupa ruler Miwang Drakpa Gyaltsen and his younger brother Sonam Gyaltsen. At this period of Tibetan history, prior to the appearance of the Dalai Lamas, Tibet was under Pakmo Drupa administration and the royal family was formally linked to that sect of the Kargyupa school. They were great patrons of Tsongkhapa, sponsoring his construction of Ganden Monastery near Lhasa, and also his institution of the Monlam Chenmo, or Great Prayer Festival of Lhasa, which was to become an annual national event. The circumstances of his writing are given in the colophon:

> This treatise on the profound path of the Six Yogas of Naropa, entitled *A Book of Three Inspirations*, was written at the repeated requests of the lordly Miwang Drakpa Gyaltsen and Chojey Sonam Gyaltsen, who asked for a work that would clarify the key points in the inner heat yogas, as well as briefly touch upon the common and exclusive distinctions in the trainings.

Tsongkhapa was in a unique position to write authoritatively on the subject. As a young monk student he had studied in forty-five different monasteries representing over a dozen sects, and thus had received exposure to an array of traditions of the Six Yogas as maintained in the various hermitages. In particular, he had received extensive guidance in the traditions preserved in the Pakmo Drupa (Kargyu), Drikung (Kargyu) and Zhalu schools. In addition, he had received numerous other lineages descending from Marpa Lotsawa, who had brought the Six Yogas to Tibet, and thus was able to bring his knowledge of these into his presentation.

Throughout his treatise Tsongkhapa quotes freely from earlier masters, and most of these quotations are derived from the Tibetan translations of early Indian works, either an original tantra or an authoritative Indian treatise. This quality pervades the pages of the hundred or so principal books that he penned. When he does quote a Tibetan lama, it is usually one of the early lineage masters belonging to the period in which the tradition moved from India to Tibet.[10]

There are a number of ways of explaining the title of Tsongkhapa's treatise, *A Book of Three Inspirations*. One of these is given in *Notes on A Book of Three Inspirations* by Jey Sherab Gyatso, who quotes the following verse from the closing section of Tsongkhapa's text in which Tsongkhapa is commenting upon the basic focus that he adopted in his composition:

> It contains clear instructions on the stages of meditation in this
>   path,
> A clear and critical guide to the principles in the trainings,
> And references to the authoritative tantras and commentaries;
> These are the three features within which it is set.

Jey Sherab Gyatso then states, "These are probably the three inspirations referred to in the title." In other words, because the treatise has these three features, it can be regarded as an object of confidence and inspiration. The same was said by the Dalai Lama's late Junior Tutor, Kyabjey Trijang Rinpochey, in his 1973 public reading of Tsongkhapa's text in Dharamsala.

A second explanation of the title of the text is given by Ngulchu Dharmabhadra in *An Ornament for A Book of Three Inspirations* and was quoted above. Ngulchu links Tsongkhapa's threefold division of Naropa's Six Yogas into "foundation, actual body and auxiliary practices" to the Indian sources from which the six are drawn. He mentions this three times in different contexts in his commentary. His reading is based on the words with which Tsongkhapa presents his sources in his Epilogue. The idea is that the substance of the first of the three, "inner heat, the foundation...," is sourced in Krishnacharya's transmissions known as *The Drop of Springtime* and *The Sambhuta Drop of Springtime*, both of which were received by Tilopa and represent the essence of the Hevajra Tantra and the Heruka Chakrasamvara Tantra teachings on *chandali*, or inner heat. The second of the three, i.e., the main body of the path, or the illusory body and clear light doctrines, represent the essence of the Guhyasamaja Tantra as expressed in the Nagarjuna tradition known as the "Arya Cycle" and embodied in Nagarjuna's *Pancha krama,* or *Five Stages.* Finally, Marpa Lotsawa had spent three years in Nepal on his first journey to India, during which he mastered the Four Seats Tantra, or Shri Chaturpitha Tantra, the source of the third of the above three categories, i.e., "the auxiliary trainings" of consciousness transference and forceful projection. Ngulchu states, "Because each of the three branches of the Six Yogas is based on such authoritative sources, Tsongkhapa entitles his treatise on the tradition *A Book of Three Inspirations.*"

SECTION ONE OF TSONGKHAPA'S TEXT

Naropa's Six Yogas belong to the category of tantric doctrine known as highest yoga tantra, and within that category they belong to the second stage of practice, which is also known as the completion stage. Thus their instructions are addressed to those who have completed the basic trainings and, as the classical expression goes, "accomplished the preliminaries."

Tsongkhapa opens his treatise, *A Book of Three Inspirations,* by dividing his presentation into two main sections: the first dealing with the preliminaries and prerequisites of entering into practice of Naropa's Six Yogas, together with a presentation of the general principles of the generation and completion stage scenarios; and the second dealing with the actual Six Yogas themselves.

The Preliminary Trainings Associated with the General Mahayana

Tsongkhapa classifies the preliminary trainings that are necessary in order to prepare one's mind for the practice of the Six Yogas as being twofold: the "common" preliminaries, and the "exclusive" ones. He then goes on to point out that the former of these refers to the general philosophical and contemplative traditions derived from the Sutrayana, or "public discourse" teachings of the Buddha. These are the general Mahayana techniques of basic observation meditation, working with karmic law, the contemplations on love and compassion, the altruistic aspiration, and so forth. Tsongkhapa does not give much space to these in his commentary, for, as he puts it, he has "written extensively on these elsewhere." Presumably by this he is referring to his *Lam Rim Chenmo,* or *Great Exposition of the Stages on the Path.*

In closing this section, Tsongkhapa drops us a gem of advice from the melodious voice of the poet and yogi Milarepa,

> If one does not contemplate the nature of karmic law—
> How good and negative deeds produce according results—
> The subtle power of the ripening nature of activity
> May bring a rebirth of unbearable suffering.
> Cultivate mindfulness of action and its result.
>
> If one does not observe the faults of sensual indulgence
> And from within oneself reverse grasping at it,
> One will not become freed from the prison of samsara.
> Cultivate the mind that sees all as an illusion
> And apply an antidote to the source of suffering.
>
> If one is unable to show kindness to every living being
> Of the six realms, who once was one's own kind parent,
> One falls into the limitations of a narrow way.
> Therefore cultivate the universal bodhimind
> That looks on all beings with great concern and caring.

Jey Sherab Gyatso in *Notes on A Book of Three Inspirations* comments that Tsongkhapa at this point in his treatise first invokes the name of Atisha Dipamkara Shrijnana, the Indian master who came to Tibet in 1042 at royal invitation and from whose work the Kadampa school (Tib. *bKa' gdams ring lugs*) emerged, and then invokes the name of Milarepa, an early lineage master in the Six Yogas transmission, in order to demonstrate that the attitudes of these two eleventh-century masters were in harmony on the need for using the general Mahayana trainings as a basis for and preliminary to tantric training.

Jey Sherab Gyatso goes on to point out that Atisha's *Lamp for the Path to Enlightenment* (Skt. *Bodhipathapradipa*) categorizes all the general Mahayana practices into three branches: initial, which involves contemplating karmic law, impermanence and so forth, in order to turn the mind away from grasping at the ephemeral things of this life and toward higher spiritual aspirations; intermediate, which involves contemplating the shortcomings of indulgence and higher worldly accomplishments, and invoking the aspiration to achieve nirvana; and vast, which involves contemplating love, compassion, universal responsibility, and the bodhisattva resolve, and giving rise to the aspiration toward omniscient Buddhahood. He then states that the three verses of Milarepa quoted by Tsongkhapa respectively embody these three steps in training.

The General Tantric Preliminaries

Tsongkhapa now turns to the "exclusive" preliminaries. Here he says, "These are of two types: the general Vajrayana preliminaries; and the preliminaries emphasized in this Naropa system."

The first of these reminds the reader that there are certain guidelines common to all Vajrayana, or tantric systems. Anyone wishing to practice the Six Yogas of Naropa, a tantric system, would therefore have to fulfill these.

Essentially there are two guidelines common to all tantric systems. The first is that the trainee must receive the tantric initiations appropriate to the system to be undertaken; second, he or she must become firmly established in the tantric *samaya*, or "sacred oaths."

The receiving of initiation from a living lineage master is regarded as an indispensable prerequisite. Tsongkhapa quotes an Indian classic, *The Mark of the Great Seal* (Skt. *Mahamudra tilika*),

> When should trainees be given instruction?
> Only after they have received the empowerments;
> For at that time they become appropriate vessels
> To receive the tantric teachings.
> Without empowerment there will be no attainment,
> Just as oil does not come from pressing sand.

The emphasis in tantric Buddhism on transmission as living tradition is thus made plain. Tsongkhapa relates the story of the first meeting between Milarepa and his disciple Gampopa. Milarepa was the direct disciple of Marpa, who in turn had received the Six Yogas directly from Naropa; and Gampopa was destined to become Milarepa's greatest disciple, as well as the forefather of all twelve Kargyu schools. Tsongkhapa writes,

> When Venerable Milarepa first met his disciple Chojey Gampopa, the former asked the latter, "Have you received the tantric initiations?" Gampopa replied, "I have received them from Maryul Loden, a disciple of Zangkar." Milarepa therefore accepted to teach him.

Maryul Loden had received the Chakrasamvara initiations brought to Tibet by Zangkar Lotsawa, a translator of Western Tibet whose name is derived from the area of his birth, i.e., Zanskar (near present-day Ladakh). Gampopa had thus received the appropriate empowerments, and consequently Milarepa could give the Six Yogas transmission to him without any other preparation being required.

Tsongkhapa concludes the section by saying, "It is best if here the empowerment is into a mandala from either the Hevajra or Chakra-samvara cycles. These two have a special connection [with the Naropa Six Yogas system]." Although these lineages were brought to Tibet by Marpa, along with the lineage of the Six Yogas, they also existed in the Land of Snows prior to Marpa's time, for example, in the lineage of Maryul Loden mentioned above.

Tsongkhapa's point is that although the Six Yogas are a synthesis of elements from diverse tantric sources, their foundation is the first of them, the doctrine of the inner heat yoga. In turn, the inner heat doctrine is drawn from two sources, namely, the Hevajra and Chakra-samvara tantric cycles. Because the inner heat doctrine is identical in the two systems, initiation into either system is valid as a basis for practicing the Six Yogas. Tsongkhapa then proceeds to discuss the various lines of transmission that he considers to be the most authoritative.

Concerning the Vajrayana preliminary of cultivating stability in the tantric *samaya*, Tsongkhapa does not elucidate the particular disciplines that are expected of a tantric initiate. These may be found, however, in Ngulchu Dharmabhadra's commentary, *An Ornament for A Book of Three Inspirations*:

> The tantric *samaya* are of three types: those concerned with eating; those concerning what is to be maintained; and those concerning what is to be owned. The first of these categories refers to eating the five meats and five nectars, and to first consecrating whatever one consumes. The second refers to the general *samaya* of the Five Tathagatas, the fourteen root and eight secondary precepts, and the nineteen individual guidelines. One should understand these four categories, as well as what constitutes a small or intermediate breach of them, and make the effort to maintain them.... As for the third category, which concerns what is to be owned, this refers to keeping a vajra and bell, the hand drum, a special mantra rosary, the bone ornaments, and so forth. One should own the actual tantric implements and objects, or else a drawing of them.... Whenever failings occur, one should respond as though a poison had been accidentally eaten and quickly apply an antidote, such as the mantra recitations and meditations of Vajrasattva or Samayavajra, the Vajradaka fire rite, and so forth.

As the Thirteenth Dalai Lama points out in "A Guide to the Buddhist Tantras,"[11] the list of fourteen root tantric vows was created by the Indian master Acharya Ashvaghosha (ca. fifth century C.E.) by drawing from a large number of early tantric treatises, and the list of eight secondary tantric precepts was compiled by Nagarjuna in his later life (ca. sixth century). Thus the tradition of "root and secondary tantric precepts" does not originate directly from the tantras taught by the Buddha, but rather is an innovation of the Indian masters Ashvaghosha and Nagarjuna.

His Holiness the present Dalai Lama comments in *Cultivating a Daily Meditation*[12] that there really are only two tantric precepts: (1) always to cultivate the vision of "radiant appearance," i.e., of the world as a mandala and oneself as the mandala deity; and (2) always to maintain the sense of tantric pride, i.e., the thought that oneself and all others constantly rest in enlightenment.

Tsongkhapa concludes his discussion of the topic of the disciplines by quoting a tantra from the Chakrasamvara cycle. He writes, "Also, *The Tantra of Interpenetrating Union* (Skt. *Shri samayoga tantra*) states,

> Not to have been introduced into the mandala,
> To ignore the tantric precepts...
> To practice on that basis produces no attainment."

The Tantric Preliminaries Unique to the Six Yogas System

The preliminaries that are exclusive to the Six Yogas legacy are comprised of two principal practices: the meditation and mantra recitation of Vajrasattva; and the practice of guru yoga, which includes the mandala offering symbolic of the universe. Tsongkhapa explains these two in considerable detail, pointing out that both of these practices are also done in other tantric systems. It is the manner in which they are performed in the Six Yogas system that makes them unique. Jey Sherab Gyatso explains their importance in *Notes on A Book of Three Inspirations*:

> The two exclusive preliminaries emphasized in the Six Yogas system are those of Vajrasattva and guru yoga. Both of these use some form of the seven-limbed devotion. Actually, from within the range of practices for purifying the mind that are common to both the general Mahayana and Vajrayana, that known as the seven-limbed devotional offering, together with the mandala offering, is predominant. Furthermore, as a means of facilitating the guarding of the Vajrayana disciplines and guidelines, the Vajrasattva meditation and recitation of the hundred-syllable mantra are recommended. And even though some manuals on the tantric trainings state that the Vajrasattva practice is unnecessary for those who keep their disciplines well, nonetheless every school and sect that

maintains a tradition of the Six Yogas of Naropa recommends it. As well, it is used in conjunction with almost all tantric systems of completion stage yoga.

What is unique in the Six Yogas system is the tradition of how the Vajrasattva and Guru Yoga practices are done in retreat or semi-retreat as five sets of 100,000. These are comprised of 100,000 refuge mantras, 100,000 physical prostrations, 100,000 mandala offerings, 100,000 Vajrasattva mantras, and 100,000 guru mantras. Other tantric systems use these same meditations, but do so as short preliminaries to each individual meditation session, or at least once a day, rather than as major retreat practices.

The tradition of doing "the 500,000 preliminaries" was introduced into Tibet by Marpa Lotsawa, and soon became standard in most schools of Tibetan Buddhism. Similarly, the legacy of a "great retreat" of three years, three months and three days was also designed by Marpa, and these days is maintained in most schools.

In my translation of *A Book of Three Inspirations* I have taken the liberty of moving Tsongkhapa's treatment of these two meditations— Vajrasattva and Guru Yoga—from their placement in the treatise to the back of the book, where they appear respectively as Appendices I and II. Tsongkhapa presents the two meditations in detail, because in his time they were not especially widespread practices, and he wanted to make it clear that he endorsed them wholeheartedly. However, due to the culturally bound nature of their language, I felt that they would distract the Western reader from an appreciation of the flow of ideas in Tsongkhapa's work.

The Generation Stage Yogas

When the above preliminary practices have been completed, Tsongkhapa recommends that the trainee engage in the generation stage trainings, which means the meditations on the mandala and its deities. He discusses the tradition of and need for the generation stage meditations as a condition for entering into the Six Yogas, all of which are completion stage yogas. He also discusses which tantric mandalas are best used for the generation stage practice, and provides us with guidelines on how the practice is best pursued. Tsongkhapa recommends meditation upon the mandalas of either Hevajra or Heruka Chakrasamvara as the basis of the generation stage training. He then proceeds to explain how one approaches and pursues the practice, whichever mandala is used.

Jey Sherab Gyatso's *Notes on A Book of Three Inspirations* speaks of how the generation stage practice centers around the process of "taking the three occasions as the path of the three kayas," which, as we saw earlier, introduces the trainee to the process of the "nine blendings." He also mentions some distinctions between how the generation stage is practiced in the Gelukpa school and how it is approached in the older schools:

> The principle behind the generation stage yogas is the process known as "taking birth, death and bardo as the path of the three kayas." By means of the generation stage yogas [the trainee] is introduced to the process of transforming the experiences of birth, death and bardo into the three kayas of enlightenment: Dharmakaya, Sambhogakaya and Nirmanakaya. This prepares the mind for the methods of the completion stage yogas, which bring about this actual transformation.
>
> The Sakya and Kargyu schools mostly rely upon simplified mandalas that use only a pair of central deities, male and female in union, such as Hevajra and consort Nairatmya, for accomplishing this ripening process of the generation stage. However, Tsongkhapa recommends that in the beginning we should practice with a complete mandala, and then later, when stability has been attained, reduce it to the central male-and-female-in-union deity. This is less problematic. He does not recommend that we use a simplified mandala from the beginning. The important principle here is that the meditation upon the supporting mandala purifies perception of the world, and meditation upon the supported mandala deities purifies the practitioner's five psychophysical aggregates.
>
> This can be accomplished by meditation upon any of a number of mandalas, but the mandala should be at least as complex as that of the Ghantapada lineage of the Chakrasamvara mandala, which has five deities, for we want to purify the five psycho-physical aggregates and transform the five inner distortions into the five wisdoms.
>
> An exception to this rule [of a mandala having a minimum of five deities], as Tsongkhapa points out in several of his writings, is the mandala of Solitary Vajrabhairava [i.e., Yamantaka], wherein a single mandala deity suffices for the process. Many lamas from other schools question Tsongkhapa's logic on this recommendation of Solitary Vajrabhairava. Tsongkhapa's idea here is that the Vajrabhairava system combines elements from both the male tantras and the female tantras, and therefore is adequate.
>
> In brief, because Naropa's Six Yogas embodies elements from both the male and female tantras, it is acceptable to practice the generation stage yogas by utilizing the mandalas from any of the

three main tantric cycles: Guhyasamaja, Heruka Chakrasamvara, or Vajrabhairava. Many of the early gurus [in the Six Yogas lineage] used either Hevajra or Chakrasamvara as their personal meditational deity, and thus accomplished the generation stage yogas in conjunction with a mandala from one of those two cycles.

Jey Sherab Gyatso then states that regardless of the mandala one uses for the generation stage yogas, it is best if one receives an initiation into either Hevajra or Heruka Chakrasamvara prior to engaging in the actual practice of the Six Yogas, which are completion stage trainings, and that the single most appropriate is that of any of the four families of Hevajra. It is obvious from Tsongkhapa's tone that a number of his readers will have heard of practicing the Six Yogas without first having undergone sufficient training in the generation stage meditations. He invokes the words of great masters of the past, and also presents his own reasoning on the topic, in order to demonstrate why he thinks such an approach is unwise. He then sums up the essence of the generation stage training most wonderfully as follows:

> From the very beginning of the generation stage yogas these two aspects of practice—divine pride and the radiant appearance of the mandala—should be cultivated as complementary. When our meditation on the supported mandala deities and supporting mandala achieves maturity, the mere mindfulness of the radiantly present image will give rise to a wonderful sense of being, in which the ordinary appearances of things do not arise. Thus the technique has the power to purify from within the mind the mundane presence of the conventional world. Similarly, if one can generate a strong sense of unfeigned divine pride as explained earlier, this will have the power to purify from within the mind the habit of apprehending things as mundane.
>
> One arises from formal meditation and goes about daily activities, seeing the manifestations of world and living beings as mandala and tantric deities. This is the samadhi that transforms the world and its living beings into a most extraordinary vision. This is what is meant by the expression, "The generation stage yogas purify mundane appearance and apprehension."

Jey Sherab Gyatso's commentary also succinctly presents the two principal elements in the generation stage yogas: radiant appearance and divine pride. He adds a note on the second of these which I have not seen elsewhere:

> The process of the generation stage yogas begins by concentrating on oneself as the lord of the mandala, surrounded by the

mandala entourage. If the central deity has many faces and hands, one first concentrates on the main face and accomplishes clarity with it. One then concentrates on the two main hands. After that one gradually supplements the visualization with other details of the main deity, and then goes on to the consort, entourage, and supporting mandala, until all appears with total clarity.

One must cultivate two principal factors: the radiant appearance of oneself as the mandala deity and the world as mandala; and the divine pride, the strong thought "I am the tantric deity."

At first this thought is contrived, but gradually it arises spontaneously. On the generation stage of practice the divine tantric pride of the form of the deity is accomplished. Then during the completion stage yoga, at the phase of practice known as "the vajra recitation," the divine tantric pride of the speech of the deity is accomplished. Finally, the divine tantric pride of the mind of the deity is accomplished at the stage of the clear light yogas.

Introduction to the Nature of the Mind

After discussing the general Mahayana and exclusively tantric preliminaries, our author then embarks upon a discussion of the general principles of the completion stage tantric yogas as the spiritual environment within which the Six Yogas will be engaged.

This begins with a discussion of "the nature of the basis," which refers to introducing the trainee to the tantric vision of the body and mind. The nature of the mind is taught first, for this awareness is of fundamental importance to the application of the tantric yogas. Here the topic of discussion is the doctrine of emptiness, for it is the rich dynamic of the emptiness of the mind and mental experiences, with its implications for the processes of perception and knowledge, that renders the spiritual process possible.

Tsongkhapa's treatment of the topic of the nature of the mind opens with a verse from Lama Marpa on how he had trained in the emptiness doctrine:

> I travelled east to the banks of the Ganges River
> And there, through the kindness of Guru Maitripa,
> Realized the uncreated nature of phenomena.
> I seized with my bare hands the emptiness nature of my mind,
> Beheld the primordial essence beyond concepts,
> Directly encountered the mother of the three kayas,
> And severed the net of my confusion.

The trademark of Tsongkhapa's approach to the subject of emptiness, the final nature of being, is his commitment to the Madhyamaka, or

"Middle View" schools of classical India. It is significant here that he presents a reference by Marpa to Maitripa, because from among Marpa's various Indian gurus, Maitripa was the master most committed to the Madhyamaka approach.

Marpa had studied with approximately fifty Indian and Nepali gurus; but the three principal ones were Naropa, Jnanagarbha and Maitripa. From the first he received, among other things, the Six Yogas; from the second he received a transmission of the Guhyasamaja Tantra, which, as Tsongkhapa points out elsewhere in *A Book of Three Inspirations*, Marpa used to adorn the illusory body and clear light doctrines received from Naropa; and from the third he received his training in the emptiness doctrine, by means of which he achieved his mahamudra realization, or understanding of the emptiness teaching.

Tsongkhapa then quotes another direct disciple of Maitripa, the illustrious Sahajavajra, who wrote a commentary to Maitripa's *Ten Reflections on Simple Suchness* (Skt. *Tattva dashaka*). Sahajavajra states,

> One should rely upon the approach to emptiness elucidated by the great Madhyamaka masters Arya Nagarjuna, Aryadeva, Chandrakirti, and so forth, who teach that the interdependent, co-existent nature of phenomena points to the suchness of being. One should adopt the guidelines set forth by these three masters.

These are Tsongkhapa's great philosophical heroes: Nagarjuna, Aryadeva and Chandrakirti. The first two are the early forefathers of the Madhyamaka movement in second- and third-century India; the third was a later elucidator of their thought.

In the centuries between Nagarjuna's early work and the advent of Chandrakirti, the Madhyamaka school had branched out into a number of different directions. Chandrakirti's famous text *A Guide to the Middle View* (Skt. *Madhyamaka avatara*) became a landmark in classical Indian Buddhist philosophy, analyzing and assessing the various philosophical trends into which the Madhyamaka schools had evolved. The Madhyamaka lineage that emerged from Chandrakirti's clarification of Nagarjuna's teachings became known as the Prasangika. Tsongkhapa regards Maitripa as one of eleventh-century India's greatest spokespersons of the emptiness doctrine that had been transmitted and clarified by Nagarjuna, Aryadeva and Chandrakirti, and as one of the greatest later Indian representatives of the Madhyamaka Prasangika view. Therefore Marpa's reference to Maitripa serves Tsongkhapa's purposes well, allowing him to address the subject of the ultimate nature of the mind with the language of the Madhyamaka Prasangika school. The salient point in Tsong-khapa's approach to the tantras is that in regard to the view of emptiness he always keeps within Madhyamaka parameters.

He summarizes the essence of the Madhyamaka message by quoting a treatise by Arya Nagarjuna entitled *The Sixty Stanzas on the Nature of Emptiness* (Skt. *Yukti shashtika*),

> All the various objects of experience
> Are like the moon reflected in water—
> Neither really true nor really false.
> Those appreciating this do not lose the view.

Tsongkhapa then continues,

> One should understand the emptiness doctrine in the context of this simile. The wise perceive that all things—persons and phenomena—arise in reliance upon their own causes and conditions, and that based on this process we impute mental labels upon things. The phenomena themselves have no true or inherent existence from their own side. They have no self-nature whatsoever....
>
> Although all things lack even the smallest speck of true existence, nonetheless conventionally the laws of causes and conditions operate through them, and conventionally all the phenomena in samsara and nirvana seem to exist, arising in the same manner as do illusions, dreams and a reflected image.

The discussion of the real nature of the mind concludes with some verses from Milarepa, Marpa's great yogi disciple, to demonstrate that Milarepa had also upheld the Madhyamaka view of Maitripa, and consequently of Nagarjuna. Milarepa sang,

> Eh-ma! Yet if there are no living beings, how then
> Could the buddhas of the three times come into being?
> Without a cause, there can be no effect.
>
> From the perspective of conventional reality,
> All things in samsara and nirvana,
> Which the Buddha has accepted as conventionally valid,
> All existents, things, appearances, non-existents,
> All these functional realities, are inseparably
> Of one taste with the quintessential nature of emptiness.
> There is no self-awareness, and no other-awareness.
> All share in the vastness of *yuganaddha*, the great union.
>
> The wise who realize this truth
> No longer see mind, but only wisdom-mind.
> They no longer see living beings, only buddhas.
> They no longer see phenomena, only the quintessential nature.

Here again Jey Sherab Gyatso in his *Notes on A Book of Three Inspirations* elaborates Tsongkhapa's position:

> These days in Tibet there are many lamas who teach that the emptiness philosophy of the tantras is different from that of Arya Nagarjuna, and that the former is higher. However, many different sources, including the collection of texts known as "Four Interwoven Treatises" (*'Grel pa bzhi sbrags*), reveal how the two systems are in harmony.
>
> Some Kargyupas even say that the mahamudra philosophy of Marpa and Milarepa is higher than the Madhyamaka emptiness doctrine of Nagarjuna. To show that the two are parallel, [Tsongkhapa] quotes a song by Lama Marpa.... This demonstrates how Marpa achieved his understanding of the mahamudra doctrine under Maitripa. This master was definitely a follower of Chandrakirti, the great elucidator of Nagarjuna's doctrine of emptiness, as demonstrated by [Maitripa's treatise] *Ten Reflections on Simple Emptiness*. [Tsongkhapa then also quotes] Milarepa...to show how Milarepa upheld this same view. So let's face it: If Marpa and Milarepa, the two great early Tibetan masters of the Six Yogas tradition, did not know the special features of the mahamudra emptiness philosophy associated with the transmission, who does? As Tsongkhapa so elegantly suggests, to take the mahamudra doctrine beyond what Marpa and Milarepa taught is to contradict the very basis of this Kargyupa legacy.

Jey Sherab Gyatso then explains why the subject of the real nature of the mind is discussed in relation to the emptiness philosophy of Nagarjuna, Aryadeva, Chandrakirti, Maitripa, Marpa and Milarepa. As he puts it, it is this most subtle dimension of the mind—the dimension which has, by means of the emptiness training, transcended its coarse obscurations of grasping at sensory phenomena as real, as well as the six or twenty-six emotional and cognitive distortions— that has the capacity to directly experience final emptiness, the ultimate nature of being. It is also this dimension of consciousness focused upon the ultimate nature of being that is implied by the term *mahamudra* as used in Gelukpa highest yoga tantra literature.

Introduction to the Nature of the Body

In the technology described by the completion stage yogas, to which the Six Yogas belong, the body and mind exist on three planes simultaneously. A different frequency of consciousness arises from each of the three physical bases. These three, with both body and mind, are simply called "coarse," "subtle" and "very subtle."

The coarse body refers to our ordinary physical presence characterized by flesh, bones and sensory powers. This "coarse body" gives rise to "coarse consciousness," the state of awareness in which conventional sensory data are processed, together with the associated intellectual and emotional dimensions of the sensory experience.

The "subtle body," also called the "vajra body," supports the "subtle consciousness." This subtle body is comprised of the network of the abiding energy channels (Skt. *nadi*; Tib. *rtsa*), the energy centers (Skt. *chakra*; Tib. *rtsa 'khor*), the flowing subtle energies (Skt. *vayu* or *prana*; Tib. *rlung*), and the emplaced sexual drops (Skt. *bindu*; Tib. *thig le*). The completion stage yogas of all highest yoga tantra systems involve working with these chakras, nadis and so forth, and therefore in all systems there is a description of how to visualize these energy factors within the body, how to bring the energies under control, and so forth. Tsongkhapa explains this process later in his text, under the presentation of the inner heat yoga.

As Tsongkhapa states in his text, the completion stage yogas of all highest yoga tantra systems speak of separating the coarse levels of the body from the subtle. In effect, the coarse are sedated by means of the tantric yogas and meditations, allowing the subtle to dominate. This in turn allows the subtle consciousness to manifest.

One persists in the tantric yogas, and eventually the very subtle body emerges. This "body" is the subtle energy that arises from the mansion created by assembling the subtle drops inside the chakra at the heart. These form into a single drop supporting the subtle physical energies, and all ordinary links with the body are severed.

When this "body" has been separated from the two earlier ones, one experiences "very subtle consciousness." The frequency of the consciousness that arises when only the heart-drop is present as the support of the energies is what is referred to as "the most subtle mind."

Gyalwa Wensapa summarizes the tantric theory of these three dimensions of body and mind very succinctly in *A Source of Every Realization: The Stamp of the Six Yogas of Naropa*:

> The body is threefold: coarse, subtle, and very subtle. The "coarse body" is the ordinary body, made of flesh, blood and bone, and born from the sperm and ovum of our parents. The "subtle body" refers to the abiding energy channels, the flowing energies, and the emplaced red and white [i.e., female and male] creative drops. The "very subtle body" is the subtle energy that supports the consciousness of the four emptinesses, especially the fourth emptiness, called "utter emptiness," which is the clear light mind....

As for the mind, it also has these three dimensions. The "coarse mind" refers to that co-emergent with the five sensory consciousnesses. The "subtle mind" is that co-emergent with the driving force of the six root distortions, the twenty secondary distortions, and the eighty conceptual mindsets. The "very subtle mind" is the dimension of consciousness that is in the same nature as the four emptinesses, and especially the fourth, "utter emptiness," the clear light mind.

A major aim of the completion stage yogas is to separate these three sheaths of the body, thus separating the frequency of the consciousness that arises from the physical bases. In this way the meditator achieves an increasingly subtle inner meditative environment.

This technology of radically refining the physical base in order to refine the state of consciousness is thus effected in two quantum leaps. This is one of the principal reasons that the tantric path is referred to as the quick path to enlightenment. The more subtle the physical base during meditation, the more subtle will be the consciousness that arises; and the more subtle the consciousness that applies a given spiritual technique, the more powerful that method becomes. This is the underlying tenet of the maha-anuttara-yoga tantras.

The Physical Exercises and Meditations upon the Empty Shell Body

Tsongkhapa recommends that, before entering into the actual practice of the Six Yogas, we engage firstly in the special physical exercises and then in the meditation upon the body as an empty shell.

The purpose of doing these as a preparation for each meditation session upon the Six Yogas is given slightly later in Tsongkhapa's text:

> When we meditate on the chakras, it is sometimes difficult solely by means of gentle preparatory methods to induce a state of samadhi having the ability to control the vital energies and to open the energy channels. When these more forceful preliminaries are done, there is less chance of undesirable side-effects occurring.

The tradition of physical exercises associated with the Six Yogas of Naropa is significant, and is one of the few examples of hatha yoga being practiced by the Tibetans. It spread from the Six Yogas lineage into other tantric traditions in Tibet.

Some manuals on the Six Yogas system speak of large numbers of different exercises. For example, the manual of Pema Karpo, the twenty-fourth patriarch of the Drukpa Kargyu school, lists the possible numbers of the different physical exercises that can be adopted as "...six, ten, twenty or fifty."[13] Also, Jey Sherab Gyatso states in his *Notes*,

> There are a wide variety of traditions on the physical exercises associated with the Six Yogas of Naropa, such as the set of six, the set of thirty-two, and so forth. The Pakmo Drupa and Drikung Kargyu schools both maintain a tradition of 108 exercises.... However, there seems to be no great advantage in doing more than the six recommended by glorious Pakmo Drupa.

Here the six recommended by Pakmo Drupa are the same as the six included by Tsongkhapa in *A Book of Three Inspirations*, for Tsongkhapa generally follows Pakmo Drupa on such technicalities throughout his treatise. Tsongkhapa describes these in some detail, but we should remember that the verbal description of each is not sufficient to convey the exact practice to the trainee. Traditionally these are physically demonstrated by the teacher when the disciple arrives at the appropriate stage in training.

These exercises are practiced in conjunction with the meditations on the body as an empty shell. Tsongkhapa describes this process as follows,

> One commences as before with the practice of visualizing oneself as the mandala deity. The special application here is to concentrate on the body, from the tip of the head to the soles of the feet, as being utterly empty of material substance, like an empty transparent balloon filled with light.

The purpose of doing these two together—the physical exercises and the empty body—is also stated by Jey Sherab Gyatso in his *Notes*:

> If one enters into the completion stage yogas [such as the Six Yogas of Naropa] without first achieving great stability in the generation stage yogas, there is the danger that one will experience considerable physical pain as a result of the changing energy flows. To avoid this, one should do as many of the physical exercises as possible, in conjunction with the meditation on the body as an empty shell. When stability in these practices is achieved, one will experience a sense of subtle joy that pervades the body, and the possibility of pain arising in the body or mind will be eliminated. When progress in the practice comes without pain or hardship, this indicates that one is proceeding correctly.

Having prepared the groundwork in this way, Tsongkhapa now introduces the subject of how the actual Six Yogas are to be practiced. Thus the remainder of his treatise is dedicated to the treatment of the individual Six Yogas.

SECTION TWO OF TSONGKHAPA'S TEXT

Tsongkhapa the Great structures the Six Yogas of Naropa as follows: (1) the inner heat, (2) the illusory body, (3) clear light, (4) consciousness transference, (5) forceful projection, and (6) the bardo yoga. As he points out, the bardo yoga is presented together with the illusory body doctrine, for reasons explained later in his text. He then states that the order of the individual six as listed does not indicate that they are practiced consecutively, and that in fact most manuals do not explain them in this order.

Two yogas not separately mentioned above as being among the Six Yogas, but which are included within them, are those of dream and sleep. Tsongkhapa's text speaks of "the daytime practice" and "the sleeping practice." The latter includes both dream and sleep yogas. As he explains, most manuals on Naropa's Six Yogas place the explanation of dream yoga in the section on the illusory body doctrine, and place the explanation of sleep yoga in the section on the clear light doctrine. Consequently, because the illusory body doctrine is generally presented in manuals prior to the presentation of the clear light doctrine, dream yoga often ends up being taught before sleep yoga. However, in the actual training one would have to become proficient in meditating on the clear light of sleep before succeeding in the dream yogas.

The idea behind the structure of the Six Yogas system as arranged by Tsongkhapa, at least the three of them that fall under the categories of "foundation" and "actual path" as mentioned above, is that the inner heat yoga (the foundation) is used to bring the subtle energies into the central channel, melt the subtle drops, and give rise to the tantric blisses. The overwhelming physical ecstasy thus invoked, said in tantric scriptures to be a hundred times more intense than ordinary sexual orgasm, gives rise to a special state of consciousness. This is focused in meditation on emptiness, the ultimate nature of being, and the ecstasy conjoined with the wisdom of emptiness emerges. This state of mind is the trademark of highest yoga tantra, and therefore of the Six Yogas tradition, and it is this to which the term *mahamudra* refers in Gelukpa tantric literature. This "ecstasy conjoined with (the wisdom of) emptiness" is the force then used to embark upon the "actual path," i.e., the illusory body and clear light practices.

Tsongkhapa is very direct on the importance of establishing this ecstasy conjoined with the wisdom of emptiness as the inner basis:

> In general, all systems of highest yoga tantra's completion stage involve the preliminary process of controlling the vital energies flowing through the two side channels, *rasana* and *lalana*, and redirecting them into the central channel. This is indispensable.
>
> There are numerous means for accomplishing this, based on the traditions of the Indian mahasiddhas, who drew from the various tantric systems. In this tradition [i.e., the Six Yogas of Naropa] the main technique is to arouse the inner heat at the navel chakra, the "wheel of emanation," and then through controlling the life energies by means of the *AH*-stroke mantric syllable, to draw the subtle life-sustaining energies into the central channel. When these energies enter the central channel the four blisses are induced, and one cultivates meditation on the basis of these in such a way as to give rise to the innate wisdom of mahamudra.
>
> Otherwise, if one does not rely upon a profound path of this nature [i.e., in which the basis of the meditation is not the innate ecstasy conjoined with wisdom awareness], but instead engages a samadhi that merely maintains a state of non-conceptual absorption for a prolonged period of time, no great signs of progress will be produced.

To illustrate the point, he refers to the first meeting between Milarepa and Gampopa, in which Milarepa asked about Gampopa's meditation. Gampopa replied that he could sit in meditative absorption for many days at a time without distraction. Milarepa told him, "You cannot get oil by crushing sand. The practice of *samadhi* is not sufficient in and of itself. You should learn my system of inner heat yoga...." The implication is that the innate ecstasy conjoined with wisdom awareness, which is aroused by the inner heat yoga, was absent, and thus Gampopa's samadhi lacked real tantric power. Arousing that "real tantric power" is the purpose and territory of the inner heat doctrine.

The Inner Heat Yoga

The purpose of the inner heat doctrine is to bring the energies into the central channel at the heart chakra, melt the "drops" and give rise to the special tantric ecstasy. This bliss is then utilized in extraordinary ways.

The Sanskrit term for inner heat is *chandali*, which the Tibetans translated as *tummo* (Tib. *gTum mo*). It is a feminine noun, with the sense of both fierceness and heat.[14] In the Six Yogas system, wherein the *chandali* practice is derived from the Hevajra and Chakrasamvara tantric cycles, this power of inner heat is symbolized by the mantric syllable known in Tibetan as *ah tung* (Tib. *a thung*), or "the short *AH*," a Sanskrit participle somewhat resembling the exclamation mark in English, or, as Ngulchu Dharmabhadra puts it in *An Ornament for A Book of Three Inspirations*, "somewhat like an upright thorn." In other words, it resembles a toothpick standing up on its thicker end. Chogyam Trungpa refers to this Sanskrit participle as "the *AH*-stroke."[15] It is always visualized in its Sanskrit form, in contrast to the practice used by Tibetans with almost all other mantric syllables of visualizing them in their Tibetan forms.

As Tsongkhapa points out, there are three principal elements involved in the meditations for igniting the inner heat: meditating on the channels; meditating on the mantric syllables; and meditating in conjunction with the vase breathing technique.

In the first of these the three energy channels are envisioned as running up the center of the body, with the chakras at the four upper sites: crown, throat, heart and just below the navel. One can also visualize four lower chakras, beginning at the navel and going down to the tip of the jewel. Beginners generally work primarily with the four upper chakras, and most texts on the Six Yogas do not give much detail on the four lower ones.

In the second step of the inner heat yoga, a mantric syllable is placed at the center of each chakra. Here Tsongkhapa gives the advice,

> Moreover, one should concentrate on the syllables of the upper three chakras for just a short period of time, and then dedicate most of the session to meditating on the *AH*-stroke at the navel chakra.

Jey Sherab Gyatso clarifies this point in his commentary, and addresses the topic of the dangers that arise through incorrect practice:

> There is no one standard way of engaging in the inner heat yoga. For example, the size in which the energy channels are visualized varies in accordance with the capacities of trainees. Similarly, the chakra recommended as the site at which to draw the energies into the central channel varies. However, there is less danger of undesirable side-effects when one works with the chakra at the navel. Consequently the two side channels are generally

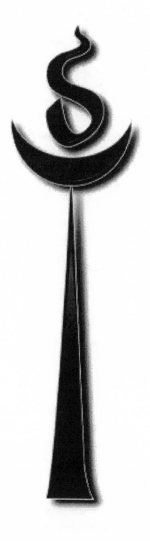

The AH-stroke syllable

visualized as curling into the mouth of the central channel at the site of the navel chakra. It is best to firstly establish control over the subtle energies at the navel chakra. Should one try to do this at any of the three upper chakras and apply the techniques forcefully, there is the danger that the upper energies will be disturbed and that negative side-effects will be produced, such as intense turbulence of the heart energies, and so forth. Similar dangers are associated with working with the secret chakra. There are numerous ways of visualizing the mantric syllables in the practice of the inner heat, as well as of retaining the energies, and in how the inner heat that is induced behaves.

In the third step, one engages in the exercises of breath control and retention in order to intensify concentration and redirect the vital energies.

Tsongkhapa elaborates these techniques as follows,

Meditating like this on the inner heat yoga has the purpose of inducing the four blisses. To effect this, first the bodhimind substance in the channels must be melted, and together with the vital energies must be brought to the chakra at the crown. This generates the first bliss, known simply as "bliss." The substances in the channels again flow, and then collect at the chakra at the throat; the second bliss, known as "supreme bliss," is aroused. Again the substances flow, and then collect at the chakra at the heart; the third bliss, known as "special bliss," arises. Fourthly, the energies collect at the chakra at the navel; the bliss known as "innate bliss" is induced.

He cautions,

The bodhimind substance that resides in the upper chakra is melted and brought to each of the four chakras, where it must be retained. If one cannot hold it in the chakras for a prolonged period of time one will not be able to appreciate the uniqueness of each of the four experiences of bliss. In particular, one will not be able to discern the uniqueness of the fourth, the innate bliss.

He then speaks of how one manipulates the subtle energies in order to cause them to enter into, abide, and dissolve within the central channel. The nature of the language in this part of the text could perhaps be called tantric psycho-speak. The ideas reflected here of the interwoven nature of the body and mind, and the relationship between the mind and the body's subtle structures of "channels," "winds," and "drops" that must be "melted and brought to the heart," are fundamental to the Vajrayana. Learned tomes have been written by Western scholars on the psychological, spiritual and biophysical implications of the chakra system; and all of this is useful in helping Occidentals get a grip on what is being talked about in the tantric process. However, traditional tantric literature prefers to maintain a language strongly characterized by multidimensional ambiguity, where the process is presented by symbol and flow rather than being reduced to a static verbal concept.

Thus Tsongkhapa can quite easily say,

> The earth energies dissolve into those of water, and the mirage-like sign is beheld; the water energies dissolve into those of fire, and there is the sign of smoke; the fire energies dissolve into those of wind, and the sign of sparks, like flickering fireflies, appears. Then the energy that carries conceptual thought dissolves into mind, and there is an appearance like that of the light of a butterlamp undisturbed by wind.
>
> It is said that the strength of the experiences indicated by these signs will eventually carry one to the stage wherein the realization of mahamudra is achieved.

On the one hand the language is very earthy, speaking of what seem to be merely the coarse elemental dissolutions. The result is realization of mahamudra, the highest wisdom. Suddenly in the space of a sentence we have jumped from the mundane to the super-transcendental.

In this way the inner heat is used in order to withdraw the coarse energies into the subtle, and to melt the drops, thus refining the basis from which consciousness arises. Tsongkhapa sums up the dynamics of the process,

> As explained earlier in the description of the descending process, the bodhimind substance is melted and arrives at the chakra at the tip of the jewel. If one can retain it without ejaculation, the innate ecstasy will be aroused. At that time one must engage mindfulness of the view of emptiness to be ascertained, and must place the mind firmly there. Rest within the inseparable ecstasy and [wisdom of] emptiness. Even if you do not have a profound understanding of the emptiness doctrine, at least avoid all distractions and rest in the singular ecstasy of the experience until the absorption becomes stable, mixing this with the beyond-conceptuality consciousness.
>
> While doing this, retain the bodhimind substance in the jewel chakra for some time. Then reverse it, bringing it back up to the crown chakra. This gives rise to the "rising-from-below" innate

wisdom. Identify this clearly in the awareness, and then fix the mind in the sphere of ecstasy conjoined with [the wisdom of] emptiness. If this is impossible, then simply try to rest the mind in the ecstasy and to blend this with the beyond-conceptuality consciousness. Remain in that state for as long as possible. This is the manner in which one cultivates the experience during formal meditation sessions.

As for how to cultivate the training during the post-meditation periods, one should note that in general merely the presence of the innate ecstasy in meditation does not mean that the realization will automatically carry over into the post-meditation periods. The ecstasy that was experienced will not necessarily become manifest in the objects that appear during everyday activities. That by itself is not enough. During the post-meditation periods one must consciously cultivate mindfulness of the experience of ecstasy and emptiness, and stamp all objects and events that appear and occur with the seal of this ecstasy and emptiness. This application causes a special ecstasy to be ignited, which one should foster.

The nature of the physical heat generated by the practice has attracted considerable attention from Western medical and scientific circles. In Tibet the culmination of a three-year retreat would often see the testing of the graduating yogis. This test was conducted by putting wet sheets over the shoulders of the naked yogis, at sub-zero temperatures, and seeing who could dry the most sheets in a given time period. Clinical experiments conducted by Dr. Herbert Benson of Harvard University on some yogis chosen by the Dalai Lama for the purpose showed the yogis easily raising their external body temperatures by up to fifteen degrees within a few moments of concentration.[16] Tsongkhapa speaks of this extraordinary side-effect of the training,

> The inner heat that can be aroused is of various types. For example, there is the inner heat in the central channel, that is first aroused in the chakras at the navel and secret place, and there is the inner heat that blazes and increases outside the central channel. Secondly, there is the heat that is aroused from the depth of the body, and also the heat aroused at the surface, between the skin and flesh. Then there is the heat [that seems to pervade] narrow [areas of the body], and the heat that seems to pervade large areas, as aroused on initial stages of practice. Then there is the heat that rises slowly, and the heat that arises quickly. Also, there is the heat that seems thick, and the heat that seems thin. In each of these pairs, the first is better than the second. The second indicates an inferior experience.

A Western vipasyana meditator once commented to me that the inner heat yogas were very important to the Tibetans, due to Tibet's cold climate, but that they weren't as relevant to Westerners, whose houses have central heating. What he failed to appreciate is that the physical heat is just a side-effect of the practice, and not the purpose or function of it. The inner heat doctrine is engaged in order to gain control over the subtle bodily energies and chemical processes, as a means of melting the drops and giving rise to the tantric blisses. This ecstasy then acts as the rocket fuel of the tantric space adventure. Control over the physical processes, such as the heating functions, are encompassed by the process, but are not the primary aim of it. As Tsongkhapa points out, this control over the subtle bodily processes, and the ability to direct the subtle energies and drops that it brings with it, comprise an indispensable foundation of all highest yoga practice. Arousing this control is the essential purpose of the inner heat doctrine.

Karmamudra

Tsongkhapa concludes his section on the inner heat doctrine with a discussion of the all-important *karmamudra*, the "action seal." This refers to the tantric tradition of sexual practice with a consort. Karmamudra in this context refers to an actual sexual partner.

The early masters in the Six Yogas lineage placed great emphasis on karmamudra practice. Marpa Lotsawa spoke of the doctrine as one of his four most treasured instructions. In Milarepa's enumeration of the Six Yogas quoted by Tsongkhapa, karmamudra practice is listed separately as one of the six. Ngulchu Dharmabhadra also mentions an alternative structure of the Six Yogas given by Tsongkhapa, a structure that lists karmamudra as one of the Six Yogas, and relegates the bardo yoga to the status of a branch of the illusory body doctrine.

However, in the system as transmitted by Gampopa to Pakmo Drupa, the karmamudra yoga is not taught separately; rather, it is presented as a branch of the inner heat yoga. Because Tsongkhapa's treatise follows the tradition of Pakmo Drupa, it does the same.

The reason for linking the inner heat and karmamudra yogas in this way is elucidated in Jey Sherab Gyatso's *Notes on A Book of Three Inspirations*:

> The inner heat yoga gives rise to the simultaneously born bliss. This ecstasy then acts as a simultaneously present condition for the practice of the sexual yogas, or karmamudra. Therefore the expression "inner heat karmamudra" is used.

In other words, in order to successfully engage in the karmamudra practice one must have control over the bodily energies, a control that is acquired by means of the inner heat yogas. When this has been made firm and the innate bliss established, the karmamudra practice is applied in order to make the quantum leap from the stage of inner heat yoga to that of the illusory body yoga.

The need for engaging in karmamudra practice in connection with inner heat yoga is explained by Ngulchu Dharmabhadra in his treatise on the Six Yogas, *An Ornament for A Book of Three Inspirations.* Earlier we spoke about the process of separating the three dimensions of the body and mind: coarse, subtle and very subtle. The various stages of this process are spoken of as "the three refinements," the three being body refinement, energy refinement and mind refinement. The process of energy control that is the function of the inner heat yoga carries one through these "refinements."

The idea here is that most of the vital energies can be brought under control and directed into the central channel solely by means of the inner heat yogas together with the vase breathing technique. However, the "all-pervading energy" is difficult to control, and it is in order to subdue this that the practice of karmamudra is required. As Ngulchu puts it,

> Through meditating on the inner heat and gaining a basic mastery of the process, one comes near to the stage of achieving the semblant clear light and actualizing final mind refinement. The inner yogas by themselves will not be able to induce the jump to that stage; for this, the inner yoga must be supplemented with the external condition of relying upon a karmamudra, or sexual partner.

The key expression here is "final mind refinement." This is a technical term referring to the stage wherein only the all-pervading energy remains to be brought under control. Once it has been mastered, one makes the quantum leap to the accomplishment of "final mind refinement," which permits the manifestation of the illusory body. It is to cross this threshold that the yogi enters into union with a karmamudra.

It is said that most monks and nuns in Tibet did not engage in the karmamudra practice, but instead took up the sexual meditations using a *jnanamudra*, or visualized consort. Whether or not this is true, or if it is just a way of maintaining the secrecy of the practice, is a point of doubt.[17]

Tsongkhapa speaks of the qualifications required of one who would engage in the karmamudra yogas:

> Here both oneself and the mudra should be beings of highest capacity, and should have received the pure empowerments. Both should be learned in the root and branch guidelines of tantric practice, and have the ability to maintain them well. Both should be skilled in the sadhana of the mandala cycle, and mature in practicing four daily sessions of yoga.
>
> Also, they should be skilled in the sixty-four ways of sexual play as described in *A Treatise on Bliss*. They should be mature in meditation upon the doctrine of emptiness; be experienced in the techniques for inducing the four blisses in general and the innate wisdom awareness in particular; and be able to control the melted drops and prevent them from escaping outside.
>
> Such are the characteristics required of the practitioners as described in the original tantras and also in the treatises of the [Indian] mahasiddhas.

However, the karmamudra practice should not be casually engaged. As Tsongkhapa puts it,

> Those not qualified to take up the karmamudra practices should instead engage in prolonged meditation upon a jnanamudra [i.e., a visualized consort], such as the mandala dakinis Nairatmya and Vajrayogini. When the practice achieves stability and the visualization arises with total presence and radiance, one can enter into sexual union with this visualized consort and arouse the four blisses. The innate ecstasy emerges, and one unites this with [the wisdom of] emptiness, thus blending mindfulness of the view [of emptiness] with the great ecstasy. This is the experience known as ecstasy and emptiness in union.
>
> If one is unable to do this, one simply relies on ecstasy and cultivates the samadhi that rests one-pointedly within that bliss.

In fact there are four mudras upon which the yogi can rely for this aspect of the training: karmamudra, jnanamudra, mahamudra, and samayamudra. The First Dalai Lama (b. 1391) explains these as follows in his treatise on the Kalachakra system of completion stage yoga,[18]

> The first three of these give rise to the immutable ecstasy. The fourth is said to be the mudra experienced as a result of accomplishing the former three.
>
> Karmamudra is explained as a maiden possessing the physical attributes of a woman, who comes to one as a result of one's previous karma. Here there is no need to visualize the experience;

the maiden herself has the ability to induce the full experience by means of her skillful embrace.

Jnanamudra is a maiden created through the power of one's visualization.

As for the mahamudra, the images within one's own mind spontaneously arise as various consorts.... One then unites with these.

Through relying upon these three types of mudra, one is led to the experience of ecstasy. The bodhimind substances residing in the upper sites fall to the tip of the jewel, where they vibrate and transform. They are retained here and are not allowed to slip away....

If the yogi is not able to move the male and female drops of his body solely through the power of meditation, he is instructed to take up practice with a karmamudra. Because the karmamudra gives him the power to direct the vital substances to the tip of the jewel, she is called "the maiden who bestows the falling ecstasy"....

The yogis...are of three types: sharp, middling and dull. The first of these rely exclusively upon mahamudra. They are able to experience the immutable ecstasy solely through union with her. The second must rely upon a visualized jnanamudra in order to generate a basis of ecstasy through which they are able to enter into the mahamudra experience. Thirdly, those of dull capacity, not having the strength or purity of mind, must rely upon a karmamudra until they gain experience of great ecstasy. Only then can they proceed to the mahamudra.

This passage occurs within the context of the Kalachakra system, which varies considerably from the Hevajra and Chakrasamvara tantric cycles upon which the inner heat doctrine of the Six Yogas is based. Nonetheless it does succinctly explain the purpose of training with a karmamudra at this point in the process, and the characteristics of the practitioner who should rely upon a karmamudra.

Ngulchu Dharmabhadra's *An Ornament for A Book of Three Inspirations* provides us with some detail on the types of karmamudras that are considered to be appropriate partners for the sexual yogas, as taught in the Indian treatises on the practice:

The types of mudras upon which one should rely are classified in various ways.

For example, they are spoken of as being fourfold in dependence upon their caste: mole-bearing outcasts; courtesan dancers, flower sellers, and washerwomen.

They are also spoken of as being fourfold in accordance with the shape of their lower aperture: lotus-like, conch-like, antelope-like, and elephant-like. Here the lotus-like is best. They are threefold in dependence upon their realization. In this context they are known as mantra-born, place-born and innately born.

The mantra-born mudra refers to an ordinary female who has purified her mind by means of the general Mahayana trainings, received the complete tantric initiations, and maintained the tantric precepts and guidelines. On those foundations she has become fluent and skilled in the generation stage yogas, and has achieved realization of the initial stages of the completion stage yogas, thus becoming a yogini born from mantra realization.

The place-born mudra is one who resides in one of the sacred tantric sites, such as any of the twenty-four Heruka sites and so forth. As for the innately born mudra, this refers to a yogini who abides in union with the clear light realization.

When both a qualified relier and a relied-upon practitioner take up the activity of meditating within the environment of sexual union, they can use the experience to cause the vital energies to enter, abide and dissolve within the central channel. The drop is brought to the jewel chakra and retained there without being allowed to leave. The melting and blisses are induced, and these are used to propel the meditator through the stages of final mind refinement.

Gelukpa literature tends to be somewhat discreet in its discussion of the topic of karmamudra practice due to the sect's emphasis upon monastic purity. As a consequence, much of the knowledge on the subject remains solely within the oral transmission. This should not be taken to mean that the practice is not honored or maintained within the Gelukpa tradition, but rather that the secrecy of the practice is stressed.

The subject of karmamudra practice is introduced to the trainee for the first time at this point in the inner heat yoga. It will continue to re-appear in the remaining practices of the Six Yogas, where it will be used to propel the trainee from the top of one stage of realization to the beginning of the subsequent stage.

The Illusory Body Yoga

Tsongkhapa begins his treatment of the illusory body doctrine with a discussion of the term "illusory body" as it is used in the Guhyasamaja system, from which the topic is derived for the Six Yogas. He also discusses how this compares to the manner in which most oral transmissions of the Six Yogas present the subject. He is not particularly impressed by the standard presentation and obviously prefers the greater sophistication of the original Guhyasamaja system.

The Guhyasamaja tradition speaks of the yogas of "body refinement," "speech refinement," and "mind refinement." These respectively refer to the process of separating the three aspects of form, energy and awareness—coarse, subtle and very subtle—from one another. The illusory body is produced on the basis of the third of these three physical dimensions. That it to say, one can only manifest the illusory body on the basis of having established "body, speech and mind refinement." If the illusory body doctrine is to be engaged as an actual highest yoga tantra practice, that must be its basis.

There is also a discussion of two levels of this illusory body: unpurified and purified. The former is known as "the illusory body of the third stage" and the latter as "the illusory body of the fifth stage." The former is concomitant with the attainment of arya status; the latter is what arises as the Rupakaya in final enlightenment.

In Tsongkhapa's opinion, many transmissions of the Six Yogas overly simplify their presentation of the illusory body, and most of them fail to appreciate these quintessential principles of the Guhyasamaja doctrine. As he puts it,

> These are the principles on which the illusory body doctrine [of Lama Marpa's tradition of Guhyasamaja] is based; but we do not see them discussed in this tradition.
>
> Instead there is a discussion of an unpurified illusory body that is linked to the practice of observing one's image reflected in a mirror as a means of cutting off the coarse conceptual mind, such as thoughts of pleasure or displeasure at likes and dislikes. Then there is a discussion of a purified illusory body, which is linked to the practice of meditating upon the illusory nature of one's own body envisioned as that of a mandala deity, which induces a state of one-tasteness that does not discriminate between likes and dislikes.
>
> Yet these two ["unpurified" and "purified" as described above] are only "illusory bodies" in a general sense common to both highest tantra and other paths. They are to be distinguished from the "unpurified illusory body" that is the third stage [of the Guhyasamaja five-stage system], known as "the hidden essence of illusory nature"; and the "purified illusory body" that is the fifth stage, also known as "the illusory body of the stage of great unification." It seems that this distinction is not even roughly made here.
>
> The actual illusory body is exclusive to highest yoga tantra. The first "illusory body" described above [i.e., observing one's image in a mirror, etc.] does not even really qualify as a general-nature illusory essence; and the second one [i.e., meditating on the illusory nature of oneself as a mandala deity] is also found in the three lower classes of tantras [and hence is not even exclusive to highest yoga tantra].

Following Tsongkhapa's guidelines, Gyalwa Wensapa describes the manner of implementing the illusory body doctrine in *A Source of Every Realization: The Stamp of the Six Yogas of Naropa*:

> After applying oneself to the technology for directing the vital energies into the central channel, one eventually achieves a mature meditative absorption fluent in the process. Soon one perceives the signs of approaching the stage wherein the illusory body can be produced.
>
> From within the sphere of sexually uniting with a karmamudra, which is the outer supporting condition, one engages the inner supporting condition, which refers to meditating on the channels, chakras, and so forth; and meditating upon the blazing and melting. The vital energies are caused to enter into the central channel, and to abide and dissolve, giving rise to the signs of the dissolutions, from the mirage and so forth until the sign of the clear light. The four emptinesses emerge in the nature of the four blisses. When the innate clear light arises, one meditates upon ecstasy conjoined with emptiness. This is the technology for engaging the innate semblant clear light, with which the basis of the illusory body is produced.
>
> When the time comes to emerge from the clear light, one arouses the instinct to set aside one's old aggregates, and to take the form of a Buddha Vajradhara, male and female in union. Then as one arises from the clear light, the vital energy of the five radiances, upon which rides the innate semblant clear light, serves as the substantial cause; and the mind itself serves as the simultaneously present condition. Based upon these, the old aggregates are bypassed, and one arises in the form of a Buddha Vajradhara, male and female in union, adorned by the marks and signs of perfection. This is the stage of the "unpurified illusory body." Simultaneously one experiences the dissolution process in reverse, going from clear light to proximate attainment, and so forth, until the sign of the mirage.
>
> In systems such as the Guhyasamaja Tantra this illusory body is illustrated and explained by using twelve similes.
>
> At that time three factors occur simultaneously: the cessation of the innate semblance [i.e., the "semblant" or "metaphoric" clear light consciousness]; the fulfillment of proximate attainment in the dissolution process; and arisal in the actual form of an "unpurified illusory body."

Tsongkhapa comments that his criticism of the treatment of the illusory body doctrines in most oral transmissions of the Six Yogas lineages applies equally to the doctrines of clear light and *yuganaddha*, or "great union." He feels that many of his contemporaries would do well to read up on the Guhyasamaja tantric literature and thus achieve an understanding of the basics. He does not mince his words on this theme,

> As had been pointed out earlier, the doctrines of the illusory body and clear light yoga have their source in the Guhyasamaja Tantra. According to the oral tradition of this tantric system coming from Arya [Nagarjuna] and his disciples, a transmission known as the "Arya Cycle," for as long as the vital energies have not been drawn into the central channel and caused to abide and dissolve, one will not be able to generate the samadhi of the threefold experience of "appearance, proximity and proximate attainment" associated with the accomplishment of mind refinement; and it is only from the state of vital energies and consciousness that have generated the complete signs of the wisdom awareness of mind refinement that the qualified illusory body yoga can be engaged.

In the Six Yogas system the illusory body training is divided into three aspects: training in seeing the illusory nature of "appearances," which encompasses everything that we experience in waking life; training in awareness of the illusory nature of dreams; and training in the illusory nature of the bardo. Thus here again we see the "three bardo states" discussed earlier.

In the first of these, one channels the vital energies into the heart chakra, and gives rise to the experience of the elemental dissolutions, until the great ecstasy and the clear light consciousness arise. This is then focused in meditation upon emptiness. In post-meditation periods one brings this "ecstasy and emptiness" into one's everyday experience. As Tsongkhapa puts it,

> During meditation sessions one invokes the great ecstasy, uses this as the driving force in the focus upon the view of emptiness, and then rests single-pointedly within that absorption of beyond-conceptuality mind. Between sessions one cultivates the awareness of how emptiness and conventional interdependent existence complement one another.
>
> In this way the two [formal sessions and between-session trainings] are applied in rotation as complementary to and supportive of one another.

This section of the text contains some of Tsongkhapa's finest expressions of his approach to emptiness; for meditation upon emptiness here is integral to the application. He writes,

This awareness of emptiness is simply an appreciation of the primordial non-inherently abiding nature of things. It is not a mental fabrication. Nor is it a partial emptiness that [is the nature of merely some phenomena and] does not pervade all objects of knowledge. By placing one's awareness on this final mode of being, all the forces that eliminate the syndrome of grasping at an "I" are strengthened.

The next aspect of the illusory body training involves working with the dream state. In the actual application of dream yoga it is necessary to borrow the technology from the clear light doctrine related to meditating on and retaining the clear light of sleep; for although a small degree of dream yoga can be implemented on the basis of conscious resolution conjoined with a conventional meditational technique, such as shamata or vipasyana, the degree of proficiency required in the Six Yogas emanates from the foundation, the inner heat doctrine, and what the meditator has achieved by means of it in terms of the yogic ability to induce the elemental dissolutions and consciously experience the stages of that dissolution, from the vision of the mirage up to the emergence of the clear light.

The ability to induce these dissolutions and retain them at their various phases during waking state meditation is instrumental to the application of the technology at the time of sleep and dream. Tsongkhapa points this out again and again. When the ability is present in the waking state, implementing it in sleep and dream is a simple matter. As he puts it,

> In the first of these... during the waking state one gathers the vital energies into the central channel and dissolves them, inducing the experiences of the four emptinesses. The manner of the application is that in the process of first retaining the clear light of sleep one cultivates awareness of the four emptinesses of sleep. After that, when dreams occur one recognizes them as such. When awareness of the four emptinesses of sleep is present, no other technique for retention of awareness in dreams is required.

The methods of implementing the dream yoga for those not having competence in retaining the clear light in meditation is explained in detail in *A Book of Three Inspirations*. Tsongkhapa elucidates the theory of sleep and dream manipulation by means of the chakra technology: which chakras to work with if sleep is too light or too thick; which energies to re-adjust when dreams are too obscure or intense, and so forth. The study of dreams is a new science in the West; for tantric Buddhists, it is an ancient art. Tsongkhapa comments,

> If one performs the above practice at the throat chakra at dusk or after dawn and still one is not able to retain one's dreams, this indicates that the practitioner is a person who naturally sleeps very deeply. To somewhat lighten the nature of sleep one should place the mind on the crown chakra.
>
> If in turn this causes one to be unable to sleep, or to sleep fitfully, then concentrate instead on the drop at the secret place. Here during the daytime one cultivates resolution as described earlier, and works with the chakra at the tip of the jewel. Before going to sleep one visualizes there a dark drop, and unites the vital energies twenty-one times [through vase breathing]. Within that sphere, and without letting the mind stray, one drops off to sleep.
>
> Sometimes working with the upper sites causes one's sleep to become too light. If this occurs, one should keep in mind that the chakra at the jewel is also associated with the sleep state, and therefore placing the mind on it will affect the depth of one's sleep. One must know how to work with the different chakras at dusk and dawn in this way in order to bring the elements [i.e., the drops within the chakras] into balance.

The dream yoga begins with cultivating the ability to retain dreams, which means the ability to recognize the dream as a dream while dreaming, without disturbing the flow of the content of the experience. In other words, one cultivates the technology of meditating throughout the sleep process, firstly absorbed in the clear-light-of-sleep meditation, and later, when dreams begin to occur, absorbed in dream yoga.

Tsongkhapa elucidates the main obstacles to be overcome in achieving progress in the endeavor, and the principal techniques involved in the application. He then deals with the methods of healing fears and obsessions that manifest in dreams, learning to cultivate out-of-body experiences in sleep, and so forth.

The Bardo Yoga

In the Six Yogas tradition the dream and bardo yogas are usually grouped with the illusory body doctrine, as Tsongkhapa puts it, "for the sake of convenience."

The reason that it is convenient to do so is because there is a common element shared by the illusory body, dream body and bardo body. All three of these physical bases are experienced when some or all of the coarse energies have been withdrawn from the coarse body, and thus all three arise from a more subtle physical base. Also, in all three situations the coarse sensory and conceptual consciousnesses have withdrawn into a more subtle dimension of the mind. Consequently in all three instances the consciousness based on that body is somewhat subtle, as compared to ordinary waking consciousness.

Tsongkhapa explains the complementary nature of the three illusory body practices as cultivated in the three bardo states:

> ...previously [one had gained proficiency] in the yogas of the clear light of sleep and of arising in the illusory body of the dream state. Familiarity with this technique causes the strength of one's illusory body practice to increase during the waking state, and that in turn supports one's practice of generating the illusory body of the dream state.
>
> Should death arrive before supreme enlightenment has been attained, and one wishes to apply the yoga for enlightenment at the time of death, then [as the death process sets in] one engages the yogas of controlling the vital energies in order to recognize the clear light of the moment of death, using the same principles that were applied in the yoga of retaining the clear light of sleep. In this way one enters into the bardo experience, applies the techniques learned through the yoga of the illusory body of dreams, and generates the bardo body as the illusory body of the bardo.

Here Tsongkhapa is establishing a link between three elements, and associating these with a kaya. There is the clear light as experienced in the waking state by means of the tantric yogas, the clear light of sleep, and the clear light of the moment of death; these are associated with the Dharmakaya. Then there is the illusory body, the dream body and the bardo body; these three are associated with the Rupakaya, in its two forms of Sambhogakaya and Nirmanakaya.

Again, to contextualize the bardo doctrine he once more refers to the Guhyasamaja tradition,

> Here the Arya Cycle of the Guhyasamaja tradition speaks of how the experience of the four emptinesses [of appearance, proximity, proximate attainment and clear light] give rise to the clear light. This is experienced much the same way as the clear light of death is experienced after the dissolution of bodily processes is complete. The yogi then produces the illusory body [by means of the four emptinesses and blisses mentioned above]; this is similar to how the bardo body is produced [after the clear light of death]. This [i.e., the illusory body] becomes the subtle Sambhogakaya,

which takes upon itself a coarse Nirmanakaya form, much in the same way that the bardo body takes rebirth with a worldly form.

A Book of Three Inspirations provides an excellent analysis of the bardo state as recorded in the Sutrayana's Abhidharma[19] literature, and then explains how this is implemented as a yoga in the highest yoga tantra systems.

As explained earlier, the Six Yogas tradition speaks of three bardo states: those of the waking state, dream state, and after-death state.

How do we proceed in the training of these three bardos? Tsongkhapa poses the question, and then offers this answer:

> Here during the waking state one practices meditation on the inner heat yoga, thus causing the vital energies to enter into the central channel, and to abide and dissolve. Through the force of this experience one induces the experiences of the four emptinesses, four blisses, and the clear light consciousness. The experience is like that of the time of death, when the vital energies and consciousnesses naturally withdraw from the body into the central channel and the clear light of death manifests.
>
> The meditations on the three clear light consciousnesses—the clear light experienced through yogic endeavor in the waking state, the clear light of sleep, and the clear light of the moment of death—are similar in that all three require that one understand the process of dissolving the vital energies and consciousnesses into the central channel just as at the moment of death, and how thus to induce the experience of the four emptinesses and four blisses.
>
> If one understands these three sets of three processes, then in the waking state application the subtle illusory body can take the form of a coarse Nirmanakaya. Also, the dream yoga can be used in the gap at the end of dreams and before waking up to cause the subtle Sambhogakaya [generated in dream yoga] to take a coarse Nirmanakaya. Similarly, after the moment of the clear light of death has passed and one enters the bardo, the same technique can be used to transform the bardo body into a Sambhogakaya form; and that in turn can be used to take a coarse Nirmanakaya form.
>
> This process is sophisticated, and one should attempt to get a clear comprehension of it. If one can gain insight into the basic principles at work in the dissolutions, then the three blendings— the clear light of death with the Dharmakaya, the bardo body with the Sambhogakaya, and the rebirth body with the Nirmanakaya— can be accomplished.

In the formal list of the Six Yogas, the bardo doctrine appears as the last of the six. However, in the order of explanation it is placed with the illusory body yoga, due to the "illusory" nature of the bardo body. As we read this section we must keep this idiosyncrasy in mind. Several topics discussed here may not make sense until one has read the next section of the book, that on the clear light, for some ideas are borrowed from that doctrine. Thus when set as the sixth and last of the Six Yogas, the bardo doctrine fits more neatly into a sequential progression: inner heat is the foundation; illusory body and clear light the main body of the path; consciousness transference and/or forceful projection branches of the path to be applied in times of emergency or in one's twilight years, in order to by-pass the bardo entirely; and, finally, if none of this works and one finds oneself entering death's gates, there is the doctrine of bardo yoga.

The Clear Light Yoga

The clear light doctrine encompasses two modes of practice: meditating upon the clear light during the waking period; and meditating upon it during sleep.

A Book of Three Inspirations speaks in depth on the various usages of the term "clear light" as it appears in the various Buddhist scriptures. Ngulchu Dharmabhadra summarizes the essence of Tsongkhapa's analysis in *An Ornament for A Book of Three Inspirations*:

> The term "clear light" is used in many different contexts: "common" and "uncommon" clear lights; the "clear light as object" and the "clear light as subject"; and the "hidden meaning clear light" and "final significance clear light."
>
> Of these, the expression "clear light as object" refers to the emptiness of all phenomena, which means the manner in which they are free from the extremes of reification and nihilism. "Clear light as subject" refers to the mind of the perceiver of that object. These usages are common to both the Hinayana and Mahayana vehicles, and to all four classes of the Mantrayana. This is also termed "the clear light of general significance."
>
> The "uncommon clear light" is a special application of the term as it appears in highest yoga tantra. It refers to the clear light as subject, wherein the "subject" is the innate great ecstasy focused in perception of clear light as object, the emptiness nature of phenomena.
>
> This highest yoga tantra usage of "clear light as subject" speaks of the clear light at the occasions of basis, path and result. Here

"clear light as basis" refers to the natural clear lights of sleep and death, and is experienced even by ordinary beings, although they do not recognize it. The "clear light of the path" refers to the semblant and actual clear lights. Because this clear light of the path is only experienced by highly trained yogis, it is also called "the hidden clear light."

Again, with the semblant clear light there is both a "proxy semblant clear light" and an "actual semblant clear light." As for the "actual clear light," there is the "actual clear light of the fourth stage" and the "actual clear light of the fifth stage." Finally, "the clear light of final significance" refers to clear light mind as experienced on the stage of *yuganaddha*, or great union. Because this state of great union has two levels, i.e., those of training and beyond training, this "clear light" is also of two types, based on those two levels of spiritual attainment.

Generating the experience of this "actual clear light" is the main purpose of highest yoga tantra. The semblant clear light is but a means to that end. A "proxy illusory body" produces the experience of the semblant clear light, and the actual illusory body produces experience of the actual clear light. This experience is most easily aroused by meditating on the inner heat at the heart chakra.

Let's examine the various usages listed by Ngulchu Dharmabhadra, beginning with the "common" and "uncommon." Here the "common clear light" refers to what is understood by "clear light" in the exoteric Mahayana and esoteric Vajrayana scriptures and in all four classes of tantras. That is to say, the usage is "common" to the various yanas. The "extraordinary clear light" refers to the exclusive usage of the term as it appears in the scriptures of highest yoga tantra.

As Ngulchu explains, the "extraordinary clear light" as used in highest yoga tantra refers to an aspect of consciousness perceiving emptiness, or "clear light as subject." The "clear light as object" simply refers to the emptiness that is the object perceived by this consciousness. Tsongkhapa points out in *A Book of Three Inspirations* that this "extraordinary clear light consciousness," otherwise known as the "clear light as subject," is invoked by meditating upon the inner heat yoga and thus giving rise to the elemental dissolutions, until the blisses are generated and the clear light mind arises. This blissful clear light mind is then retained and brought into focus on emptiness.

Ngulchu mentions "clear light as basis, path and result." The "basis clear light" is equally possessed by all living beings, from the highest to the lowest, and from the most evil to the most enlightened. The "clear light of the path" is the "basis clear light" as brought into conscious experience by means of the tantric yogas; because it is not perceived by ordinary living beings, but only by those trained in the yogas, it is also known as "the hidden clear light."

The "clear light of the path," i.e., as experienced through the tantric yogas, has many levels of realization. The two principal of these are known as "semblant" and "actual." Both of these have a "proxy" and an "actual," which refers to the manner in which the various phases of the illusory body yoga are integrated into the clear light yoga. The "semblant" is experienced on the third of the five stages leading to full enlightenment, wherein one achieves arya status; the "actual" is experienced on the fifth stage, known as *yuganaddha*, or "great union," which is the stage of final enlightenment. As Ngulchu states, this "great union" also has two stages, and thus there are two levels of the experience of the clear light consciousness associated with it.

The various levels through which practitioners evolve as they manifest the stages of realization of the illusory body and clear light are based upon the application of the inner heat yoga. Thus the inner heat is "the foundation," and the illusory body and clear light yogas are "the actual path."

Earlier we saw how these two elements—illusory body and clear light realizations—develop in reliance upon one another. The dynamics of this process, as Tsongkhapa states several times in his treatise, is lucidly explained in the Five Stages tradition of the Guhyasamaja tantric cycle. Jey Sherab Gyatso advises us in his *Notes on A Book of Three Inspirations*:

> It is important to critically examine the teachings of Lama Tsongkhapa in order to plant the instincts of realization. In particular, three of his tantric works—*A Book of Three Realizations* (Tib. *Yid ches gsum ldan*), *A Clear Lamp on the Five Stages* (Tib. *Rim lnga gsal don*), and *The Complete Seat* (Tib. *gDan rdzogs*)—should be studied in conjunction with one another. Then an inconceivable understanding is produced. This is especially important in gaining profound appreciation of the illusory body and clear light doctrines.

The first of these three texts, of course, is the treatise translated here.

Tsongkhapa divides the actual practice of the clear light doctrine as taught in the Six Yogas of Naropa into two: how to train in the waking state; and how to train in the sleep state.

Practice of the clear light yoga during the waking state essentially refers to engaging in the inner heat yoga in order to collect the vital energies into the central channel and cause them to abide and dissolve, melting the drops and giving rise to the blisses and the experience of the four emptinesses. The signs of the elemental dissolutions occur, from the mirage up to the clear light. The ecstasy of the clear light experience is conjoined with meditation upon emptiness, and the clear light is then retained. Tsongkhapa describes it as follows,

> One places the mind firmly... causing the energies from the side channels of *rasana* and *lalana* to enter, abide and dissolve within the central channel, arousing the four emptinesses, and giving rise to the amazing clear light consciousness of the path. When this occurs one observes the mind of the great innate ecstasy and then holds to it.

The application here seems to be what Evans-Wentz and Dawa-Samdup included in their *Tibetan Yoga and Secret Doctrines*[20] as "The Yoga of the Long *HUM.*" This is the absorption of the world and its inhabitants into light and then into oneself as the Samayasattva, or "Symbolic Being." This dissolves into the mantric syllable *HUM* at one's heart, which is the Jnanasattva, or Wisdom Being, the symbol of the ultimate nature of one's own mind. This in turn dissolves into light, from the bottom upward, into clear light. As the *HUM* dissolves, the stages of the dissolution process are invoked, and the according visions appear, beginning with the mirage up to the clear light. When the clear light ecstasy emerges one unites it with emptiness meditation. Thus we have the "short *AH*" (or *AH*-stroke) of the inner heat doctrine, and the "long *HUM*" of the clear light.

The training in cultivating the clear light of sleep entails a more specified application, and thus, as with the dream yoga, involves working with the different chakras in order to finely tune one's sleep patterns and bring them into harmony with what is required for the implementation of the yoga.

The principle behind the clear-light-of-sleep doctrine is described as follows in *A Book of Three Inspirations*,

> In general it is said that the drop which supports the experience of the deep sleep state naturally resides in the heart chakra. When one utilizes this as a path one can induce an amazing experience of the clear light of sleep. Even when it is not utilized as a path, the vital energies naturally withdraw into this drop when one goes to sleep. Hence if during the waking state one cultivates the ability to bring the vital energies into the central channel, and

> when going to sleep applies the meditations described above, maintaining the visualizations inside the central channel at the heart chakra, it becomes quite easy to bring the energies into the central channel at the heart....

The illusory body and clear light doctrines, powered by the inner heat application, are explained as being the main body of the path; thus they are the principal means for inducing the experience of enlightenment. Tsongkhapa points out that the manner in which these two work together is presented with greatest clarity in the Arya Cycle of Guhyasamaja doctrines, and thus this aspect of them should be gleaned from that source.

This takes us to the last two of Naropa's Six Yogas, both of which are categorized as "branches of the path," namely, consciousness transference and forceful projection.

The Consciousness Transference Yoga

The premise behind the doctrine of consciousness transference is that the state of one's body and mind at the moment of death makes a tremendous difference to the experience of dying, and to how one will enter the bardo. This affects the outcome of the bardo experience, and the subsequent rebirth.

Various techniques are taught in the Sutrayana and Mantrayana for working with this situation.[21] The technique advocated in the Six Yogas system comes from the highest yoga tantras. Its key point is that it aims to prepare the death channel by means of yogic application during one's lifetime, so that when the moment of death comes one can slip gently out of the body via this passage, and project or transfer one's consciousness to a desired rebirth, such as in a buddhafield paradise, or as a tantric practitioner in the human realm. This death channel is easily prepared by means of yogic application, especially if maturity in the inner heat, illusory body and clear light yogas has been established. However, as *A Book of Three Inspirations* states, "it is best to undertake the training when one is not weakened by disease." To prepare the death passage, one should engage in the yoga while still having full strength.

As Tsongkhapa points out, there are a wide range of consciousness transference techniques available from the different sutra and tantra sources; and, even within highest yoga tantra, a wide range of practices exist. As he puts it,

There are a number of oral tradition teachings on the subject. That known as "consciousness transference by means of the four techniques" and also the Ngok lineage of consciousness transference provide wonderfully detailed presentations of the meditations involved. However, in this tradition [i.e., the Six Yogas of Naropa], the oral transmissions of most lamas present the instructions of consciousness transference based on oral transmission alone.

He then summarizes the practice as follows,

Here the oral tradition suggests that one visualize oneself as one's mandala deity, and bring the vital energies into a kiss at either the secret place or the navel chakra. One then envisions the red *AH*-stroke syllable at the navel chakra; at the heart chakra, a dark blue *HUM*; and at the crown aperture, a white *KSHA*.

Now one pulls up forcefully on the vital energies from below. These strike the *AH*-stroke syllable at the navel chakra, which then rises and strikes the *HUM* at the heart. This rises and strikes the *KSHA* at the crown. Then the process is reversed: the *HUM* comes back down to the heart chakra; and the *AH* comes back down to the navel chakra.

Here sometimes it is said that the *AH*-stroke syllable dissolves into *HUM* [and that into the *KSHA*] during the upward movement. The approach as described above is more effective.

One should apply oneself to this training until the signs of accomplishment manifest, such as a small blister appearing on the crown of the head, a sensation of itching, and so forth.

In this way the death passage is opened. Then at the "time of actual application," which means the moment of death, one engages the same yoga as had been used to open the death passage, and exits the body consciously.

Tsongkhapa quotes from *The Diamond Sky Dancer Tantra* (Skt. *Vajradaka tantra*), in which it is said,

One purifies the limit of the residence.
Having purified it, one implements the transference.
Otherwise, there will be no benefit.

He explains that the phrase "limit of the residence" refers to the human body, the residence within which we live. He then says, "To try and engage the transference yogas without first having purified the body by means of the inner heat yoga explained earlier will produce no meaningful results." In other words, the power used to clear the death passage emanates from the inner heat application.

Tsongkhapa keeps his discussion of the consciousness transference doctrine brief; for, as he states, he has written on the subject in detail elsewhere.[22]

The Forceful Projection Yoga

Most commentaries to the Six Yogas written in the last three or four hundred years do not count forceful projection, or "drong-juk" (Tib. *grong 'jug*), as one of the six. Usually only a paragraph or line is dedicated to it, placed discretely at the conclusion of the explanation of consciousness transference. To compensate for the deletion, either karmamudra yoga or dream yoga is elevated to the status of one of the "Six Yogas" to make up the number six. The logic of deleting it is that theoretically this doctrine is no longer practiced; or, if it is, it is used only in the strictest secrecy. The usual explanation is that the practice lineage died with the mysterious death of Marpa's son Darma Dodey, to whom the lineage had been passed.

The practice itself is exotic: transferring one's consciousness into a fresh corpse. To get the hang of it, one begins by training in the technique by means of attempting to revitalize the bodies of small animals. Eventually one can work up to the real thing, a human corpse. Tsongkhapa describes in detail how the corpse is placed on a mandala table in front of oneself, and the meditations conducted. At the time of actual application one fetches a fresh corpse from the charnel ground, places it cross-legged on the table, sits facing it, and projects one's consciousness into it, thus reviving it. One then cremates one's old body, and goes on about one's business in one's new residence.

Why would one want to do such a thing? Tsongkhapa offers this answer:

> The reasons for performing forceful projection into another residence can be multifold. For example, there are those of inauspicious lineage who find that they are unable to accomplish great deeds for the benefit of the world due to physical limitations, and thus may feel it expedient to acquire a more appropriate body. Also, perhaps a physical illness renders one unable to benefit oneself or others, and therefore one is moved to acquire a healthy body. Similarly, one may be afflicted by old age and thus be moved to acquire a youthful body.

Although this all sounds a bit far-fetched, and quite rightly is included in the Six Yogas only as an auxiliary practice, the subject seems to have been of great interest to eleventh-century India and Tibet. For example, it is said that when Marpa's son, to whom the technique of forceful projection had been given, fell off his horse and was about to die, he quickly projected his consciousness into the body of a pigeon and flew away to India. There the pigeon alighted on the breast of a young boy who lay dead on a funeral pyre. Marpa's son then projected his consciousness out of the body of the temporary vehicle, the pigeon, into that of the boy. The pigeon fell over dead, and the boy sat up. He became known as Tipupa, the Pigeon Mahasiddha. A generation later Milarepa sent one of his disciples, Rechungpa, to study with Tipupa in India.

Biographies of the Indian mahasiddhas and yogis of the period are filled with such anecdotes. The tradition continued in Tibet, especially with the early Kargyupa lamas. Yogis quite casually throw their spirits into the bodies of geese, foxes or other creatures, leaving their human body behind in a state of suspended animation, and then come back some time later, exiting the borrowed body and re-entering the old aggregates. Marpa is said to have demonstrated this phenomenon several times to his disciples.

Of course, corpses for the practice were far more easily acquired in those days. Only the wealthy were cremated. Most towns and cities had a charnel ground nearby, where the dead were brought and deposited, to be offered as food to the wild animals and vultures as a final act of generosity. A yogi would have a good selection of bodies from which to choose.

These charnel grounds were favored meditation places for the Indian mahasiddhas. Usually they were located at the edge of a jungle and thus had a host of wild animals, from tigers to jackals, looking to them as a food source. Many of the mahasiddhas practiced meditation in charnel grounds. Often these were located near a city, and thus had a hefty turnover of bodies. It is said that the simultaneous presence of decomposing corpses and hungry scavengers provides an environment most conducive to tantric meditation.

A rumor concerning the doctrine of forceful projection is that originally there were two techniques: one for projection into a corpse; and another for projection into a living being. It was the second application that caused the consternation that led to the mysterious death of Marpa's son and the ostensible ending of the lineage.[23]

Tsongkhapa also mentions two applications for "drong-juk": forcefully projecting one's consciousness into a fresh corpse in order to take up residence there; and, secondly, offering one's own body to someone in need, by means of forcefully projecting their consciousness into one's body, and vacating it for them. Tsongkhapa does not say much on the subject of the second application, for, as he puts it, "This second tradition is not publicly taught by the gurus."

The qualifications of the practitioner of these branch practices are described as follows:

> With all three practices—consciousness transference, forceful projection [into a corpse], and projecting someone out of their body into one's own body—one requires the ability to block the flow of energies by placing mantric syllables at the gates, and also the ability to purify the gates by means of using the vase breathing technique to direct the vital energies into the central channel. And one needs the ability to control the red element, [symbolized by] the *AH*-stroke syllable at the navel chakra, by means of the inner heat yogas, and utilize it to arouse the consciousness that rides upon the subtle energies, represented by the *HUM* at the heart chakra.

Concluding Notes

Having elucidated the key principles in the tradition of Naropa's Six Yogas in considerable detail, Tsongkhapa wraps up his treatment with an account of how this all translates into the experience of enlightenment:

> After the stage of the great union of a trainee has been achieved one enters into meditation on the clear light, through which all instincts of the confused state of grasping at duality are washed away. Then at the time of finally manifesting the Dharmakaya, the illusory body of the practitioner on the stage of the great union of a trainee utterly transforms and becomes an illusory body of the great union beyond training. That illusory body will not falter for as long as samsara exists.
>
> At that point the clear light as an object [i.e., emptiness] possessing the two pure qualities becomes the Uncompounded Dharmakaya. The clear light as subject [i.e., as the perceiving mind] becomes what is known as the Jnana Dharmakaya, or Wisdom Truth Body, and as the Mahasukhakaya, or "Great Ecstasy Body."
>
> The support of that [Dharmakaya state] is the Rupakaya, created solely from [the most subtle levels of] energy and mind of the form-aspect of the being. This is the Sambhogakaya....
>
> Here this illusory body of the stage of the great union transforms into the Nirmanakaya, and is able to send forth countless emanations.

Gyalwa Wensapa provides a similar presentation in *A Source of Every Realization: The Stamp of the Six Yogas of Naropa*:

> The yogi on the stage of great union of training cultivates the absorptions of that level during both formal meditation and post-meditation sessions, and eventually sees signs of the approach of the attainment of great union beyond training. He engages the external condition of uniting with a karmamudra, and the internal condition of meditating single-pointedly on emptiness, causing the vital energies to enter into the central channel, and to abide and dissolve. The signs occur, beginning with the mirage and so forth, until eventually the signs of the clear light manifest. The four emptinesses arise in the nature of the four blisses.... The moment this innate clear light manifests, one engages the meditation of ecstasy conjoined with [the wisdom of] emptiness. The first moment of this clear light is the unobstructed stage on which the perceptual obscurations (Skt. *nyer avarana*; Tib. *shes sgrib*) are transcended. The second moment of it is also the first moment of omniscient buddhahood, wherein one remains in perfect absorption upon the final nature of being, while at the same time directly seeing all conventional realities as clearly as a piece of fruit held in the hand. The body of great union of training becomes the great union beyond training, the actual Sambhogakaya endowed with the kisses of the seven excellences, and that sends out thousands of Nirmanakaya emanations to benefit those to be trained. Thus one achieves complete buddhahood in the nature of the three kayas.

Tsongkhapa concludes his treatise with a summary of the early lineage, early literary sources connected with the Six Yogas tradition, and his account of why and for whom he composed the text.

THE SIX YOGAS OF NAROPA IN ENGLISH TRANSLATION

The first full translation of a Tibetan text on the Six Yogas to have been published in English seems to be that included by Lama Kazi Dawa-Samdup and W. Y. Evans-Wentz in their volume *Tibetan Yoga and Secret Doctrines*. Like all four volumes brought out by this team, the edition has the blessing of a reasonably well-qualified Tibetan lama as the translator, and the genius of Evans-Wentz as editor. The shortcoming of all four volumes is that the lama died before most of the material was published, and Evans-Wentz did not know Tibetan. Thus they were edited and annotated from his notes, and from what he could glean from diverse sources. The outcome, although not always accurate, is true to the spirit of the many texts they brought out together. Their rendition of Pema Karpo's treatise on the Naropa tradition is one of their best efforts.

Certainly the most clearly reasoned presentation of the Six Yogas in English is that provided by Herbert Guenther in *The Life and Teachings of Naropa* (Oxford, 1963). Here we have a traditional explanation of the system blended in with the story of Naropa's training under Tilopa; and then Guenther's existential analysis.

Garma C. C. Chang (also known as Chang Chen Chi), a Chinese Chan scholar, also brought out two translations, one being the treatise of Karma Tashi Namgyal, a prominent sixteenth-century writer in the Karma Kargyu school; and the other being a rough draft translation of Tsongkhapa's treatise.

The latter project began in the late 1950s, when an American scholar, Dr. C. A. Muses, acquired a number of Tibetan manuscripts, mostly initiation manuals. He hired Garma C. C. Chang to translate them, and in the process borrowed a copy of Tsongkhapa's treatise, *A Book of Three Inspirations*, from the American Library of Congress, having Chang bang out a quick translation while he was on the project.

An immediate problem was that Chang had a strong sectarian aversion for Tsongkhapa, doubtless acquired during his brief training in a small, provincial Karma Kargyu monastery in Kham, eastern Tibet. His contempt floods onto the pages of his book, especially the footnotes, in arrogant, tasteless and irrelevant remarks. To make matters worse, Chang was mostly trained in Chan, and only poorly so in Tibetan Buddhism, with no prior exposure to Gelukpa literature. Thus he was ill-equipped for the task given to him.

After completing a rough translation of Tsongkhapa's treatise, Chang had a falling-out with Muses, leaving the latter to complete the editing work. This rough draft, minus corrections and polishing, was destined for the publishers, and came out in the volume entitled *Esoteric Teachings of the Tibetan Tantras* (Falcon's Wing Press, 1961). Besides being exceedingly unpleasant in its treatment of the author whose work it translates, it contains literally hundreds of errors.

When my publishers at Snow Lion approached me with the request to prepare a decent translation of Tsongkhapa's treatise on the Six Yogas, I hesitated to accept. However, my editor asked that at least I check the Chang translation against the Tibetan original before deciding. I agreed to do so.

To compare Chang's translation with Tsongkhapa's original work I chose the sampling approach, flipping through the Tibetan loose-leaf text at random, reading a passage, and checking to see how Chang had translated the piece.

In the first passage to which I opened *A Book of Three Inspirations*, Tsongkhapa discusses the importance of gaining maturity in the generation stage yogas before going on to the completion stage applications. He quotes a verse from the *Hevajra Tantra*, wherein it is said, "Abiding equally in the two stages of tantric practice / Is the Dharma taught by Buddha Vajradhara." His point is that the generation stage yogas are an indispensable preliminary to the completion stage. Chang's translation reads, "If one says the two Yogas are equal, / It is a Dharma-infant's preaching." Goodness, I thought, that's a bit off. Either he had an edition with terrible misprints, or had been drinking heavily that night.

I flipped to a different passage, in which Tsongkhapa is in the middle of a discussion centering on the mandalas that are best adopted for the generation stage practice in conjunction with the Six Yogas. He comments,

> Thus there are these two mandalas [Hevajra and Heruka Chakra-samvara, that have been used by great lineage masters of the past]. The teaching on *tummo*, the inner heat yoga, is common to both of them. Thus either mandala practice is appropriate...

I turned to Chang's translation:

> Although there are two such transmissions (of the Luipa sixty-two deity mandala of Chakrasamvara), they both provide the methods of producing bliss and joy; therefore the practice of either one will do.

Essentially he had misread the Tibetan abbreviations of the names of the mandalas of the tantric deities Chakrasamvara and Hevajra, or *De Kyey* (Tib. *bde dgyes*), rendering them as "...bliss and joy," and thus missing the whole point of what is being said. To compensate for his confusion, he had tagged the entire passage onto what had previously been said about the Luipa transmission of the Chakrasamvara mandala, and hoped for the best. His gamble didn't work. Tsongkhapa is saying that one should use either the Hevajra or Heruka Chakrasamvara mandalas for the generation stage yogas, because the *tummo* teaching is the same in both of them; Chang has him saying that either one of the two Chakrasamvara lineages in the tradition of the Indian mahasiddha Luipa are equally appropriate because "they both provide methods of producing bliss and joy." Of course there is no tradition of speaking of two Luipa lineages of the Chakrasamvara mandala, but Chang doesn't seem to have known this.

On my third test Chang went from very bad to much worse. Tsongkhapa is discussing a number of lineages of simpler mandala practices associated with the Chakrasamvara cycle that can be adopted if one finds the Luipa tradition of Chakrasamvara or any of the four families of Hevajra to be too complicated. He states,

> The mandala should be at least as complete as that of the five-deity Heruka Chakrasamvara mandala of the Ghantapada tradition. Adopting one of the above mandalas as the basis, one engages in the practice in four daily yogic sessions.

Chang renders this as, "One should thus practice the Yoga of Four Periods which will lead to the unfoldment of the Mandalas from the feet—the Five Buddhas and Bells—to the head."

Hummm, I thought again, that's certainly very, very off. He had completely misread the name of the Indian mahasiddha whose lineage was being referred to, known in Tibetan as *Tilbu zhab* (Tib. Dril bu zhabs), or Ghantapada in Sanskrit, which literally means "Bell Feet." This really threw Chang for a loop.

Actually, the mahasiddha's name was "Bell," or "Ghanta" in Sanskrit. The "Feet" (Skt. *pada*; Tib. *zhabs*) part of the name is merely an honorific that can be tagged on to the end of almost any name. The mandala and its lineage transmission is always referred to as *Tilbu Lha Nga* (Tib. Dril bu lha lnga), or "Bell's Five Deities," Bell being the Indian mahasiddha Ghantapada, and the mandala named after him having five deities. Chang had just tossed the words in a hat, shaken them around a bit, and read them however they came out, like William Burroughs' thing with cutting up newspaper columns and then arbitrarily gluing the pieces together. It is amazing that he did not recognize Ghantapada's name, for Naropa's guru Tilopa had himself mainly practiced the generation stage yogas based on the Chakrasamvara mandala known as "Bell's Five Deities."

My next divination landed me in the introductory section of the illusory body doctrine, which in the Six Yogas system is said to be extracted from the *Guhyasamaja Tantra*. Tsongkhapa lists a dozen points of the doctrine that are not discussed in the Six Yogas transmission, but are fundamental to the process as taught in the Guhyasamaja system. The concept was obviously too much for Chang, and he simply

states, "Again, there are instructions such as given here...." He then
goes on to list as contents of the Six Yogas teaching the dozen or so
topics that Tsongkhapa is saying *aren't* discussed in the Six Yogas.

I continued with another half-dozen random samplings. Mistakes
large and small glared from the pages on each occasion.

Finally I checked the colophon. Tsongkhapa comments,

> Even though this tradition [i.e., the Six Yogas] has inspired ex-
> traordinary activities in this part of the world over the past gen-
> erations, these days the practice of it is not particularly wide-
> spread. Yet there are many people with interest in it, and there-
> fore I thought that perhaps it may be useful to accept the request
> [to write this treatise].

Chang comes up with the following,

> This book was written with the pure wish of spreading the Dharma
> of this school [Gelugpa, low school], which is thriving in this re-
> gion to a great extent; however, it has not yet reached the full-
> flourishing state.

He utterly misconstrues the passage. Why he bothers to foolishly
throw the adjectival "low school" into the text in brackets in reference to the Gelukpa is anyone's guess.

More irritating than Chang's many mistakes is his habit of continually throwing a barrage of insults at Tsongkhapa and the Gelukpa
school originating in him. For example, footnote 55 reads, "Here is
shown Tsong Khapa's 'timidness' on Shunyata, and his materialistic
view is clearly reflected." This after he has totally mistranslated the
passage he is criticizing Tsongkhapa for writing! Footnote 91/92 reads,

> These statements reflect the typical polemic and pedantic charac-
> ter of Tsong Khapa and many other Tibetan scholars, who have
> been busily engaging in controversial argumentation on trifles
> and matters of secondary importance in the past few centuries....
> Few of them had a creative mind capable of producing a new
> philosophy like the glorious teachings of Hwayan and Zen Bud-
> dhism of China.

Being a Gelukpa tantric practitioner myself, who in his youth had
practiced Zen, I was becoming a bit irritated. Perhaps terming us the
"low school" was the turning point in my reading. No one should
have to pay good money to buy a book by an author in whom they
are interested, and then have to put up with such utter silliness from
the translator. I phoned up Snow Lion and agreed to re-translate the
text for them.

In the footnotes to my translation I point out some of Chang's most serious misreadings. I have limited these to gross distortions of historical or philosophical import, as the errors number in the hundreds. However, I felt it necessary to address the most serious of them, because early translations such as his are often quoted or used as reference sources by Buddhologists not having access to the Tibetan language, and hence these mistakes get repeated.

THE SEVENTH DALAI LAMA'S *PRAYER TO THE SIX YOGAS LINEAGE*

Most Dalai Lamas have received and practiced "Naro's Six Yogas." The Second Dalai Lama (b. 1475) even wrote two treatises on the subject, one being a presentation of the tradition as a whole, and the other a summary of the principal meditation techniques involved. The Third Dalai Lama (b. 1543) wrote extensively on the five-deity mandala of the Heruka Chakrasamvara tradition of the Indian mahasiddha Tilbupa, or Ghantapada, which is the mandala most often used for the generation stage training by those embarking upon the path of the Six Yogas.

The Seventh Dalai Lama (b. 1708) received three separate transmissions of the Six Yogas of Naropa from his senior tutor Trizur Ngawang Chokden (Tib. 'Khrid zur ngag dbang mchog ldan). After the elderly guru had given the third and final transmission of the Six Yogas to the young Seventh Dalai Lama, he asked his disciple and successor to compose a prayer to the lineage masters. The Seventh, always quick to burst forth in verse, proceeded to do so. This brief poem/prayer was included in my *Selected Works of the Dalai Lama VII: Songs of Spiritual Change* (Snow Lion Publications, 1982). Here the translation has been slightly modified.

The text is in three parts: the first invokes the names of the lineage masters; the second is the prayer of the actual Six Yogas; and the third is the dedication.

As is standard with lineage prayers, the Seventh Dalai Lama gives the name of the person who served as the principal lineage holder in each generation. Readers will recognize some of the names that appear in the list prior to that of Tsongkhapa, for many of them are quoted in *A Book of Three Inspirations*, such as Naropa, Marpa, Milarepa, Gampopa, Pakmo Drupa, Drikungpa Jigten Gonpo, and so forth.

The section of the prayer dealing with "the path" follows the structure of the outlines provided in *A Book of Three Inspirations*:

preliminaries derived from the shared path, preliminaries exclusive to tantric training, the generation stage yogas, and the completion stage yoga's Six Yogas.

In this section the names of the lineage gurus are written phonetically, without formal spellings or dates. Anyone interested in such data can check the standard lineage manuals. We can presume that each master represents an average of twenty-five years of history, for each name stands for a successive generation. Milarepa was born in 1040, so this gives a rough idea of the period of each generation after him. Tsongkhapa (b. 1357) represents the twelfth generation from Milarepa, according to the chronology of the lineage given by the Seventh Dalai Lama below.

> Namo guru daka dakini yeh!
> O all-pervading Heruka and your mandala of bliss,
> O Tilopa, also known as the sublimely wise Jnanabhadra
> Who took the insight of ecstasy and void to its limits,
> And Naropa, an embodiment of Chakrasamvara:
> I request you, bestow blessings, that we may achieve
> The wisdom of ecstasy and void conjoined.
>
> O Marpa Lotsawa, a crown ornament among vajra holders,
> O Milarepa, the Laughing Vajra who gained the vajra ground,
> And Gampopa, the Doctor from Dakpo, he of the vajra family:
> I request you, bestow blessings, that we may achieve
> The wisdom of ecstasy and void conjoined.
>
> O Pakmo Drupa, great protector of living beings,
> O Drikungpa Jigten Rinchen Gonpo, a guide to the living
>   beings
> And Tsangpa Rechung, fulfiller of the needs of the world:
> I request you, bestow blessings, that we may achieve
> The wisdom of ecstasy and void conjoined.
>
> O Jampa Palwa, a master translator,
> O Sonam Wangpo, a treasury of spiritual realization,
> And Sonam Sengey, the great communicator:
> I request you, bestow blessings, that we may achieve
> The wisdom of ecstasy and void conjoined.
>
> O Yangtsewa, who saw the essence of all teachings,
> O Buton Rinchen Drup, crown ornament of the wise,
> And illustrious Khedrup Jampa Pel, learned and accomplished:
> I request you, bestow blessings, that we may achieve
> The wisdom of ecstasy and void conjoined.

O Drakpa Jangchup, who gained the Dharma eye,
O omniscient Tsongkhapa, a great king of Dharma,
And the Dharma heir Khedrup Palzangpo:
I request you, bestow blessings, that we may achieve
The wisdom of ecstasy and void conjoined.

O Jetsun Basowa, he of fabulous wisdom,
O Chokyi Dorjey, who found the ground of liberation,
And Wensapa Lobzang Dondup,[24] a most excellent spiritual
    friend:
I request you, bestow blessings, that we may achieve
The wisdom of ecstasy and void conjoined.

O Sangyey Yeshey, who destroyed all spiritual distortions,
O Lobzang Chogyen, the all-seeing [First Panchen Lama],
And Damchoe Gyaltsen, the great spiritual hermit:
I request you, bestow blessings, that we may achieve
The wisdom of ecstasy and void conjoined.

O Menkangpa, a lord of the secret yogas,
O Lama Shri, who accomplished the secret path,
And Trichen Ngawang Chokden, lord of secret doctrines:
I request you, bestow blessings, that we may achieve
The wisdom of ecstasy and void conjoined.

And I call to the mandala deities:
Heruka Chakrasamvara, in nature great ecstasy,
Vajra Varahi, the dakini who bestows the four blisses,
And the dakas and dakinis who always delight in bliss:
I request you, bestow blessings, that we may achieve
The wisdom of ecstasy and void conjoined.

Inspire us to see that life is brief as lightning, and
That all samsaric creations are in the end left behind,
So that our minds may naturally attune to spiritual ways
And may dwell in serene distaste for indulgence.

Every living being in countless past lives
Again and again has been a mother to us
And has thus suffered physically and emotionally for us.
Inspire us to arouse the sublime bodhimind,
The extraordinary compassion that seeks self-enlightenment
In order best to be able to repay their kindness;
And inspire us to untiringly pursue
The mighty ways of the bodhisattva heroes.

The spiritual teacher is the root of every siddhi;
Inspire us to cultivate an effective working relationship

With a qualified master of the tantric path,
And to cherish the disciplines as we do our very lives.

Inspire us with the Mantrayana's generation stage vision,
In which all perceptions appear as mandala and deities
And all experiences are fulfilled in skillful great bliss,
That our continuums may evolve and mature.

Vital energies generated by inner and outer means
Are drawn into *avadhuti*, the central channel,
Igniting the fires of the inner heat.
Inspire us in this yoga, that we may realize
The innately arising great ecstasy
Aroused by the touch of the secret drop.

And inspire us in the illusory body yoga:
The art of seeing all waking-state appearances as illusions;
The art of engaging the illusory body of dreams
When sleep sedates the coarse mind, the energies collect,
And the clear light of sleep emerges;
And, the art of applying the principles of the dream yoga
To the bardo at the time of death,
Thus gaining full control over all psychic emanations.

Inspire us to attain to the glory of the realization
Of the innately blissful clear light mind,
And to sculpt the primordial drop of life
Into Heruka Chakrasamvara in union with the dakini,
That in this very life the state of great union may be won.

Should our karma bring death before highest wisdom is
     achieved,
Inspire us then to confidently engage the technology
For merging mother and child clear lights as Dharmakaya,
And in the bardo to arise as Sambhogakaya
Able to send out countless Nirmanakaya emanations
In order to work for the good of the world.

Should death come before these doctrines are accomplished,
Inspire us to correctly apply the samadhi
Of consciousness transference, by directing the mind
Out of the body via the crown's golden aperture
Into *Kajou Zhing*, pure land of the dakinis;
And also inspire us to accomplish the yoga
Of forceful projection to a new residence.

May Heruka and the Yogini, as well as all dakas and dakinis,
Care for us until full enlightenment has been gained.
May their blessings pacify all negative conditions

And foster every situation conducive to growth and joy,
That we may quickly and easily cross the two stages
Of the esoteric Mantrayana path.

As with all lineage prayers associated with different lines of transmission, the verses to the early gurus are not originals by the Seventh Dalai Lama, but rather are traditional stanzas composed and handed down over the passing generations. The Seventh Dalai Lama probably just added the name of his own guru, Trichen Ngawang Chokden. The remainder of the material is, of course, his own original verse.

I checked the lineage as recorded by the Seventh Dalai Lama against those recorded in several other lineage manuals. Up to the time of Tsongkhapa and his immediate successors the list was consistent in all of them. After that there were divergences. It would seem from this that within the Gelukpa there was both a mainstream lineage of transmission, and also alternate transmissions that were preserved in various monasteries and hermitages across Central Asia.

SOME HISTORICAL LINEAGE CONSIDERATIONS

The Gelukpa attitude toward the early Kargyupa lamas is that Marpa, his four chief disciples (Lama Mey, Lama Tsur, Lama Ngokpa and Milarepa, foremost of whom was Milarepa), and Milarepa's two chief disciples, Gampopa and Rechungpa (foremost of whom was Gampopa), were flawless exponents of the tantric doctrines that Marpa had gathered in India. Of Gampopa's four main disciples, each of whom formed his own sect (known as "the four older Kargyupa schools"), Pakmo Drupa was the one to receive the most comprehensive transmission, and thus is considered to be Gampopa's principal successor. Hence he is special among the four. Tibetan historians therefore considered the Pakmo Drupa school to be the most authoritative of the four older Kargyupa schools in terms of representing the totality of Marpa's legacy.

This was the situation recorded by Tibet's greatest historian, Goe Lotsawa (b. 1392), in his masterpiece, *The Blue Annals* (Tib. *Deb ther sngon po*; trans. George Roerich, Calcutta, 1949). Goe Lotsawa relates how one day the elderly Gampopa announced that henceforth Pakmo Drupa should sit at the head of any gathering in his monastery, thus pointing him out as his principal successor.

Pakmo Drupa had eight disciples, each of whom founded a separate sect, which together are known as the "eight younger Kargyupa schools." Goe Lotsawa's *Blue Annals* states that the most comprehensive transmission was that received by Drikungpa Jigten Gonpo (also known as Jigten Sumgon) (b. 1143), the founder of the Drikung Kargyu school. Most Gelukpas agree with Goe on this, and regard the Drikung Kargyu School to be special among the eight. Thus the Pakmo Drupa sect is first among the four older Kargyupa schools, and the Drikung Kargyu first among the eight younger. Therefore the lineage that Tsongkhapa the Great recommends, as demonstrated by the lineage prayer of the Seventh Dalai Lama above, lists the early transmission masters as Tilopa, Naropa, Marpa, Gampopa, Pakmo Drupa and then Drikungpa Jigten Gonpo.

Even though Tsongkhapa the Great, the founder of the Gelukpa school, was one of Tibet's most enthusiastic, prolific and articulate commentators on the doctrinal transmissions coming from Marpa Lotsawa, who is regarded as the Tibetan forefather of the Kargyu school, relations between the Gelukpas and one of the twelve Kargyupa schools, the Karma Kargyu, rather rapidly deteriorated. Numerous scholarly papers have been dedicated to the main events of this conflict, for in the end it had far-reaching effects on Tibetan history.[25]

What is of importance to our subject of study here is that the confused history that the Gelukpa share with the Karma Kargyu has not obstructed the practice or popularity within the Gelukpa of the lineages deriving from Marpa, Milarepa and Gampopa, the early Kargyu forefathers. Marpa's Guhyasamaja transmissions have always remained central to Gelukpa doctrine throughout the centuries; and although Marpa's tradition of Naro's Six Yogas does not play as primary a role in Gelukpa doctrinal infrastructure as it does in the Kargyu schools, it nonetheless has attracted constant interest over the generations.

When Gelukpa writers comment that firstly the Pakmo Drupa Kargyupa and then the Drikung Kargyupa founders received the most authoritative transmissions of Marpa Lotsawa's lineages, this should not be taken to mean that they regard the lineages of the other ten Kargyupa schools to be inferior or less valid. These two are merely "the most complete transmissions." Tsongkhapa makes this clear in his closing comments in *A Book of Three Inspirations*,

> Marpa transmitted his lineage [of the Six Yogas of Naropa] to three of his disciples: Ngokton, Tsurton, and Milarepa. In turn, Milarepa

transmitted his lineages to two main disciples: Chojey Gampopa and Rechungpa. The lineage descending from Gampopa multiplied into many different forms, each with its own specialty, uniqueness and individual views on the different practices.

The Gelukpa attitude is that each of the twelve Kargyupa sects holds lineages that are as powerful as those of the Pakmo Drupa and Drikungpa schools in terms of having the capacity to lead trainees to enlightenment. Therefore when it is said that these two schools "received the most authoritative transmissions from Gampopa," this does not imply that they were superior in a strictly spiritual sense. The idea is that the other ten Kargyupa schools were mainly given streamlined oral tradition teachings (Tib. *man ngag*) descending from Milarepa and focusing on practice, whereas the Pakmo Drupa and Drikungpa schools received the totality of Marpa's lineages: the "practice lineages" (Tib. *sgrub brgyud*) from Milarepa, as well as the "teaching lineages" (Tib. *bshad brgyud*) from the other three of Marpa's four chief disciples (Lama Ngokpa, Lama Mey, and Lama Tsur). For Tsongkhapa, this puts the Pakmo Drupa and Drikungpa schools in something of a better position to discuss the underlying principles and philosophy of the overall transmission.

Although relations between the Karma Kargyu and Gelukpa schools have often been strained, nonetheless feelings of mutual respect have generally characterized the relationship between senior Karma Kargyupa and Gelukpa lamas over the centuries. This is wonderfully exemplified by a short song spontaneously written in praise of Tsongkhapa by the Eighth Karmapa (b. 1507), who at the time was the supreme patriarch of the Karma Kargyupa school and also a close friend of the Second Dalai Lama. At the time of the composition the Eighth Karmapa was travelling through the Charida mountains, when he experienced a vision of Tsongkhapa. He wrote:

> At a time when nearly everyone in this northern land
> Was living in utter conflict to Buddha's Way,
> Without mistake, O Tsongkhapa, you polished the teachings.
> Hence I sing this song to you, the sage of Ganden Mountain.

> When the teachings of the Nyingmapa, Kadampa, Sakyapa
> And Kargyupa schools in Tibet were in decline,
> You, O Tsongkhapa, revived the true spirit of Dharma.
> Hence I sing this song to you, the sage of Ganden Mountain.

> Manjushri, the Bodhisattva of Wisdom, gave to you
> Direct guidance in the transmissions of Nagarjuna.

O Tsongkhapa, upholder of Nagarjuna's Middle View,
I sing this song to you, the sage of Ganden Mountain.

"Mind and form are not empty of their conventional presences,
But are empty of truly existent mind and form."
O Tsongkhapa, Tibet's greatest teacher of the emptiness
    doctrine,
I sing this song to you, the sage of Ganden Mountain.

In merely a few short years you completely filled
The vast lands between China and holy India
With peerless holders of the saffron robes.
Hence I sing this song to you, the sage of Ganden Mountain.

Those who follow after you, and who
Look to you and your sublime instructions
Are never ever disappointed or mistaken.
Hence I sing this song to you, the sage of Ganden Mountain.

The trainees who follow in your footsteps
Breathe the fresh air of the Great Way.
They would sacrifice their lives to benefit the world.
Hence I sing this song to you, the sage of Ganden Mountain.

Anyone who harms your lineage must face
The terrible wrath of the Dharmapala guardians.
O Tsongkhapa, who abides in truth's power,
I sing this song to you, the sage of Ganden Mountain.

In visions and in dreams you come
To those who but once call to you.
O Tsongkhapa, who watches with compassionate eyes,
I sing this song to you, the sage of Ganden Mountain.

In order to tame humans and gods you spread
Your lineages throughout the Tibetan and Mongol regions.
O Tsongkhapa, subduer of barbarians,
I sing this song to you, the sage of Ganden Mountain.

For beings who are coarse and far from the Way,
You heal the illnesses of spiritual cloudiness, negativity and bad
    karma,
And, O Tsongkhapa, bring about quick spiritual progress.
Hence I sing this song to you, the sage of Ganden Mountain.

Those who turn to you for spiritual inspiration,
Even those of little spiritual promise in this life or the next,
O Tsongkhapa, have their every aspiration fulfilled.
Hence I sing this song to you, the sage of Ganden Mountain.

Here in Tibet you exposed the many false interpretations
Obscuring the excellent teachings given by the Buddha,

And thus firmly established your bold legacy.
Hence I sing this song to you, the sage of Ganden Mountain.

Your life embodied a sublime simplicity and discipline;
The style and fragrance of your works were incomparable.
O Tsongkhapa, gentle master most pleasing to the buddhas,
I sing this song to you, the sage of Ganden Mountain.

Through the noble deeds of the masters in your lineage,
And by the merit of this song offered to you in faith,
May the enlightenment activities of the buddhas and
    bodhisattvas
Inspire the beings of this earth for ages to come.

Something of the great Tsongkhapa's role in the transmission of the
Six Yogas lineage may be gleaned from the closing lines of Jey Sherab
Gyatso's *Notes*, where he praises the lineage of the Six Yogas and its
transmission through Tsongkhapa:

> Naropa's Six Yogas was the unique instruction of the early
> Kargyupa lamas. Lama Tsongkhapa the Great received this tradi-
> tion and later composed his treatise on the system, *A Book of Three
> Inspirations*. Thus the Six Yogas came into the Gandenpa [i.e.,
> Gelukpa] order.
>
> The Kargyupas are especially renowned for their tradition of
> the Six Yogas, and their early lineage masters, such as Marpa,
> Milarepa, Gampopa, Pakmo Drupa and Drikungpa Jigten
> Sumgon, were flawless elucidators of the tradition. However, as
> the lineage passed from generation to generation a large number
> of subtle points of confusion and error found their way into many
> of the oral transmissions. Jey Gyalwa Nyipa [the Second Buddha,
> i.e., Tsongkhapa] removed these, and clarified all the key points
> and basic principles of the system. For this reason the lineage of
> Naropa's Six Yogas as practiced within the Gelukpa order today
> is especially powerful....
>
> *A Book of Three Inspirations* is an inconceivably profound guide
> to the practice of the Six Yogas of Naropa. Even if one searches
> throughout the three worlds of existence, one would find it diffi-
> cult to discover a teaching equal to this work by Lama Tsongkhapa.

A PARTING PERSPECTIVE ON TSONGKHAPA THE GREAT

Tsongkhapa's charisma as a teacher became legendary. Tibetans love
to tell the story of his first encounter with Gyaltsab Jey (b. 1364), who
was destined to become his principal Dharma heir. At the time of
their meeting Gyaltsab Jey was a brilliant but rather arrogant monk
of the Sakya school. He had heard of Tsongkhapa's reputation as a
philosopher, and set out to challenge him to a public debate.

At the time of Gyaltsab Jey's arrival Tsongkhapa was teaching to a gathering of disciples. Gyaltsab Jey walked up to the front of the group and sat down beside the master on the teaching throne. The disciples looked on somewhat aghast, but Tsongkhapa spoke on without the slightest hesitation, and simply moved over on his seat in order to offer Gyaltsab Jey a bit more space. In the end, Gyaltsab Jey walked to the back of the crowd, prostrated, and sat down to listen. He remained with the master from that day onward, and when Tsongkhapa later passed away, in 1419, he inherited the Ganden Throne.

Tsongkhapa is sometimes portrayed in Western literature as a mere intellectual, but this view does not take into account his profound yogic accomplishments. Together with eight disciples he undertook a four-year Guhyasamaja retreat in the Olkha Mountains in order to pursue intense meditation, and a few years later spent another year in meditation retreat.[26] During the four-year retreat, he and all but two of the eight disciples who accompanied him lived on only a handful of juniper berries a day. Tsongkhapa is said to have prohibited the two elder disciples from participating in this "taking the essence" (Tib. *bcud len*) approach to eating, and insisted that, in view of their age, they take normal food.[27] He himself, and the remaining six disciples, cultivated "taking the essence," using juniper berries as the "essence pills."

Tsongkhapa lived in an intellectually vibrant period of Tibetan history, before the affliction of "political correctness" came into Tibetan thinking concerning sects and sectarianism. It was a time when lama philosophers could discuss and debate inter-sect issues without being accused of being sectarian. Gyaltsab Jey's first meeting with Tsongkhapa reflects this.

Perhaps the greatest example of this atmosphere comes in the person of one of Tsongkhapa's greatest philosophical antagonists, the Jonangpa lama Bodong Chokley Namgyal (b. 1376). This most extraordinary lama, who was also an important guru of the First Dalai Lama (b. 1391), spent half his time writing about the different Buddhist lineages of transmission in Tibet (his *Collected Works* contains over a thousand titles); the other half he spent wandering through the monasteries and hermitages of the different sects, and challenging the leading lamas to come out and debate their philosophy with him. Nobody thought him sectarian for doing so. If the monks in his targeted monastery would not consent to meet him in debate he would sit in the courtyard, read from the treatises of some of the monastery's most revered lineage masters, and chide the monks on points with which he disagreed, inviting anyone to come down and discuss the issue. His reputation intimidated many of those whom he challenged, and sometimes he would have to sit for days in the courtyard, singing songs and composing poems abusing the monks for not having the courage to defend their lineage masters.

Once he came to a monastery of the Sakya school, and the only monk who would consent to meet him was the sixteen-year-old Khedrup Jey (b. 1385). Khedrup Jey prevailed in the debate that followed, and the two became close friends. Later Khedrup Jey became one of Tsongkhapa's chief disciples. In fact, his name immediately follows that of Tsongkhapa in the lineage of the Six Yogas of Naropa, indicating that it was he who became the principal recipient of Tsongkhapa's lineage of the Six Yogas of Naropa. Moreover, after the death of Gyaltsab Jey, who had succeeded to Tsongkhapa's throne at Ganden Monastery, Khedrup Jey was installed as the Holder of the Ganden Throne.

Tsongkhapa was made of the same mettle as was Bodong. His writings freely discuss the practices, theories and philosophies of different schools. Although no mention is made of the name of the lama or school whose trend on a given topic is being criticized, any Tibetan intellectual of the period would know who was being implicated in each instance. More importantly, the lamas whose views and practices were being challenged would know that the finger was pointing at them. This wonderful, somewhat Socratic quality of fourteenth century Tibetan literature becomes increasingly rare after the seventeenth century.

Naropa's Six Yogas is an ancient legacy, with a glorious past and a strong presence in the world today. At any given time there are at least a few dozen practitioners engaged in the traditional three-year retreat focusing on the practice somewhere in the world. There are tens of thousands who have received the initiations and the transmissions, and who practice less formally. Moreover, there are millions across Central Asia who glowingly know of the system through traditional folklore and aspire to practice it, either in this lifetime or in a future one.

A Book of Three Inspirations

*A TREATISE ON THE STAGES OF TRAINING
IN THE PROFOUND PATH OF NARO'S SIX DHARMAS*

*Zab lam na ro'i chos drug gi sgo nas 'khrid pa'i rim pa yid ches
gsum ldan zhes bya ba*

by Tsongkhapa the Great,
the Buddhist monk Lobzang Drakpa

Prologue

With great reverence I pay homage to the lotus feet of my spiritual masters, who are inseparable from Buddha Vajradhara.[1]

I bow at the feet of the glorious spiritual master, who
In nature is a Buddha Vajradhara enriched in eight ways:
Body, speech, mind, miraculous ability, omnipresence,
Wish-fulfillment, excellence, and power.

The [Indian] mahasiddhas Tilopa and Naropa
Gathered the key points of the profound tantric teachings
Into the transmission known as "Naro's Six Dharmas,"
The fame of which has spread into all directions.

Having been repeatedly requested to write a commentary
   [to the Six Yogas of Naropa],
The request coming from one holding the ancestral lineage
Of a being on the exalted platform of serving as chieftain
To fortunate trainees who applied themselves to this path,[2]
I herein set forth this commentary to that profound tradition.

The explanation of the oral tradition teaching famed everywhere as "the profound path of Naro's Six Dharmas" (Tib. *Zab lam na ro chos drug*) is taught under two headings: the preliminary meditations, which build the foundations of this path; and, on the basis of those foundations, how one meditates upon the path.

The preliminary meditations, which build the foundations of this path

The preliminary meditations are of two categories: those preliminaries that are general meditations derived from the common [i.e., exoteric] Mahayana, or Great Vehicle teachings; and the preliminaries that belong to the exclusive [i.e., esoteric] Uttara-tantra-yana, or Highest Tantra Vehicle.[3]

THE PRELIMINARIES THAT ARE GENERAL MEDITATIONS DERIVED FROM THE COMMON MAHAYANA TEACHINGS

The preliminaries derived from the common Mahayana are taught under two topics: a discussion of just why it is necessary for a training in this tradition [i.e., in the tantric legacy of the Six Yogas of Naropa] to be preceded by a training in the practices of the common Mahayana; and the actual stages of training the mind in that path [i.e., in the meditations deriving from the common Mahayana teachings].

Why it is necessary for training in this tradition to be preceded by training in the practices of the common Mahayana

One certainly should train in the preliminary practices that are common to [i.e., shared by] both the [exoteric] *Paramitayana* [i.e., the common Mahayana] and the [esoteric] *Mantrayana* [i.e., the tantric vehicle].

This is clearly stated by all the principal elucidators of this lineage descending from Lama Marpa, including Lama Ngokpa, who quotes

The Hevajra Tantra in Two Sections (Skt. *Hevajra tantra nama*) as saying,[4] "Firstly impart the precepts of purification," etc., until "And after that teach the Middle View." [Lama Ngokpa] goes on to point out that this passage clearly teaches that the trainee should first be led through the practices common to both Mahayana vehicles, i.e., the ordinary Mahayana and the esoteric Mantrayana. He comments that this is the advice found in all the original tantric scriptures.

Also, it is recorded that when Venerable Milarepa taught the oral instruction transmission for achieving liberation in the bardo he said,

> First establish the basics, such as Refuge in the Three Jewels, the two aspects of the enlightenment mind—aspirational and engaged—and so forth. Otherwise both [guru and disciple] will fall over the precipice of spiritual disaster, like two oxen yoked together.

Like that, to take upon oneself the precepts [of tantric initiation] but not to guard them well will only lead both the spiritual friend [i.e., the guru] and disciple over the precipice of disaster, like two oxen tied together in one work-harness.[5] Similarly, to enter into a high tantric practice merely because of having heard of its power and beneficial effects is an invitation to disaster.

Thereafter Venerable Milarepa gave the initiation of the Yogini, and imparted the oral instructions.

The above expression "the oral instruction transmission for achieving liberation in the bardo" (Tib. *bar do 'phrang sgrol gi man ngag*) is synonymous [with the Six Yogas of Naropa]. The above manner of leading disciples [by firstly establishing them in the foundation practices] therefore applies equally to both.[6]

In particular, the Dharma master Chojey Gampopa, as evident in his work known as *Treatise on the Four Dharmas* (Tib. *Chos bzhi'i 'grel pa*),[7] strongly advises that as a preliminary [to tantric practice] one first train the mind in the stages of the path of the three spiritual perspectives. This refers to the trainings of the ordinary Mahayana.

Some manuals on the Naropa Six Yogas system, such as that by the illustrious master Pakmo Drupa, do not contain a section elucidating the preliminary practices. This is not because these lamas do not advocate the preliminaries, but because in their traditions the Naropa Six Yogas are given to disciples only after they have completed the basic trainings. These, which they call "the public teachings," are equivalent to the *Lam Rim* trainings[8] [lit., the "Stages of the Path," a term referring to the general Mahayana practices as structured by the eleventh-century Kadampa masters.]

The Six Yogas' manual of [the Drikung Kargyupa lama] Yangonpa [b. 1213] is the same in this respect, and admonishes those wishing to engage in the practice of this Naropa system to firstly train the mind well in the basic Mahayana meditations.

Thus the Six Yogas are a well-balanced transmission for guiding trainees through the quintessential practices of both the sutra and tantra paths. This is one of its great features, and we should appreciate it in this context.

The actual stages of training the mind in that path

How does one train the mind in the general preliminaries, those stages of the path that are shared by both Mahayana vehicles?

Here one should follow the advice found in the oral tradition teachings of the great Atisha [the Indian master Atisha Dipamkara Shrijnana, b. 982, forefather of the Kadampa school], wherein it is said that one should begin by cultivating an effective working relationship with a qualified spiritual master, and should dedicate oneself to him or her by means of both thought and action. On top of that one cultivates awareness of both the worth and the rarity of the precious human rebirth, and generates the firm aspiration to extract the essence of it by means of training the mind accordingly.[9]

In that entering into the Great Way is the supreme method of extracting this essence, and as the door by which one enters into the Great Way is that of giving birth to the bodhimind (Skt. *bodhichitta*)— the supreme bodhisattva aspiration to achieve highest enlightenment as a means of benefiting oneself and all others—one should give birth within one's mindstream to a pure experience of this universalist perspective. When a pure experience of the bodhimind has been induced, this signifies that indeed one has entered into the Great Way.

However, should that level of experience be mere words, then one's status as a practitioner of the Great Way is reduced to mere words. Therefore those with intelligence strive to eliminate the conditions that obstruct the birth of the bodhimind, and to cultivate an authentic experience of it.

In the beginning one must turn the mind away from grasping at the ephemeral things of this life. Not to do so only encourages obstruction to the spiritual path, be it of the Hinayana or Mahayana.

Hence one should begin by cultivating mindfulness of how this life does not last for long, how death is always close at hand, and how after death one may have to wander in the lower realms of samsara if the mind is not purified and trained in wisdom. In this way one turns the mind from grasping at the things of this ephemeral life.

Next one contemplates well the nature of the samsaric mind and the limitations of even the highest samsaric pleasures. This turns the mind from grasping at worldly glory and instead points it toward spiritual liberation.

Then, in order to turn the mind from attachment to the individual peace and joy induced through spiritual practice, one cultivates the meditations upon kindness, love, compassion, and the bodhisattva spirit characterized by universal caring. In this way one gives birth to an authentic experience of the bodhimind. One complements this with a knowledge of the ways of the bodhisattvas, and generates the aspiration to train in them.

Next, when one has confidence that one is able to carry the load of the bodhisattva ways, one takes the bodhisattva oath and adopts the general trainings in the six perfections [i.e., generosity, discipline, tolerance, joyous energy, meditative absorption and wisdom]. In particular, one cultivates both tranquil sitting (Skt. *shamatha*), which makes the mind more powerful and is in the nature of meditative absorption; and also cultivates special insight meditation (Skt. *vipasyana*), which perceives how all phenomena are like illusions and are space-like, a contemplative experience that is in the nature of the perfection of wisdom.[10]

After this, if one feels one is able to carry the responsibility of the commitments and precepts of the tantric path, one studies the text of *The Fifty Verses on the Guru* (Skt. *Guru panchashika karika*)[11] in order to understand how to cultivate correctly a relationship with a tantric master, and [applying those guidelines to one's relationship with one's own teacher] should enter into tantric practice.

If before entering into tantric practice one does not train in the preliminaries of the basic Mahayana as explained above, then one will not be able to cut off clinging to the ephemeral things of this life, and as a consequence will not experience a stable aspiration to engage in spiritual practice. Consequently one's spiritual dedication to practice will not pass beyond mere words, and the inspiration one extracts from the Three Jewels will not deeply affect one's mind. This in turn will mean that one will not experience a stable awareness of the nature of karmic cause and effect, and hence will not be inspired to maintain any of the spiritual disciplines that one has adopted.

One's practice consequently will remain superficial. One becomes unable to arouse the experience of release from samsaric addictions, and thus interest in spiritual liberation fades to intellectualization. One is unable to generate an authentic experience of the aspirational bodhimind, which is characterized by love and compassion, and consequently one's status as a Mahayanist exists in name only. An authentic aspiration to cultivate the bodhisattva ways does not arise, and hence one does not experience a solid commitment to cultivate the resolve of the engaged bodhimind. One's practice of tranquil sitting and special insight do not develop well, and one's meditative absorption lacks focus. Consequently one is unable to arouse insight into the vision of the non-self nature.

Those who want to avoid these dangers should, as a preliminary to the Six Yogas of Naropa, train the mind well in these basic Mahayana themes, the practices common to both Mahayana vehicles [i.e., shared by both the Sutrayana and Vajrayana].

The mighty Atisha, who united three lineages—that coming from Maitreya to Asanga [b. fourth c.], known as the "vast bodhisattva ways' transmission"; that coming from Manjushri to Nagarjuna [b. second c.], known as "the wisdom view transmission"; and that descending from Shantideva [b. seventh c.], known as "the transmission for exchanging self-awareness for universal awareness"— stated that these are the preliminaries to be cultivated by anyone entering into the Mahayana by the door of either the Paramitayana or Vajrayana.

Venerable Milarepa [b. 1040] put it as follows:

> If one does not contemplate the nature of karmic law—
> How good and negative deeds produce according results—
> The subtle power of the ripening nature of activity
> May bring a rebirth of unbearable suffering.
> Cultivate mindfulness of action and its result.
>
> If one does not observe the faults of sensual indulgence
> And from within oneself reverse grasping at it,
> One will not become freed from the prison of samsara.
> Cultivate the mind that sees all as an illusion
> And apply an antidote to the source of suffering.
>
> If one is unable to show kindness to every living being
> Of the six realms, who once was one's own kind parent,

One falls into the limitations of a narrow way.
Therefore cultivate the universal bodhimind,
That looks on all beings with great concern and caring.

And also, elsewhere Milarepa said,

I experienced fear at the thought of the eight bondages
And meditated on the shortcomings of impermanent samsara.
Thus I settled my mind on the objects of spiritual refuge
And learned to observe the laws of karmic cause and effect.

I trained my spirit in method, which is the bodhimind,
And cut off the stream of negative instincts and obscurations.
I learned to see whatever appears as mere illusions,
And thus no longer need fear the lower realms of misery.

Therefore, as said here, one should meditate upon these general preliminary practices until a firm inner stability has been achieved.

Gain a panoramic understanding of the complete body of the path to enlightenment, and then practice accordingly. The basis of the undertaking should be a cultivated understanding of the complete body of the path to be traversed. Then the results are extraordinary.

I have written extensively elsewhere on the practices of the general preliminary trainings, the shared path, so will not say more here.[12]

THE PRELIMINARIES THAT BELONG EXCLUSIVELY TO THE HIGHEST YOGA TANTRA TRADITION

These are of two types: the general Vajrayana preliminaries; and the preliminaries emphasized in this Naropa system.

The general Vajrayana preliminaries

The first of these—the general Vajrayana preliminaries—will be taught under two headings: showing why it is necessary to receive the complete empowerments (Skt. *abhisheka*); and showing why it is necessary to observe the tantric precepts (Skt. *samaya*).

Why it is necessary to receive the complete empowerments

In the traditions of the principal lineage holders of the tantric systems coming from Lama Marpa, including those of Lama Meton and Lama Ngokton, it is said that one should receive the four tantric initiations as a preliminary to meditating upon the two stages of the Secret Mantra Path.

When Venerable Milarepa first met his disciple Chojey Gampopa, the former asked the latter, "Have you received the tantric initiations?"

Gampopa replied, "I have received them from Maryul Loden, a disciple of Zangkar." Milarepa therefore accepted to teach him.[13]

On another occasion, before Milarepa gave Gampopa an oral transmission teaching, he sent him to receive empowerments from Bari Lotsawa.

Moreover, it was the practice of the illustrious Pakmo Drupa to insist that his disciples receive the four complete empowerments before entering into tantric practice.

All great masters of the Marpa tradition holding the oral instruction and tantric scripture transmissions unanimously agree on this. Hence it is certain that we must receive the four complete tantric initiations.

The same thing is strongly stated in the original tantric treatises [translated into Tibetan from Sanskrit]. For example, in section two of *The Mark of the Great Seal* (Skt. *Mahamudra tilika*) we read,

> When should trainees be given instruction?
> Only after they have received the empowerments,
> For at that time they become appropriate vessels
> To receive the tantric teachings.
> Without empowerment there will be no attainment,
> Just as oil does not come from pressing sand.
>
> Should a teacher out of pride in his scriptural knowledge
> Teach the secret tantric methods
> To someone who has not received the tantric empowerments,
> Both teacher and disciple immediately after death
> Certainly will fall into the hells,
> Even if some *siddhi* had been gained.
> Therefore all who strive on the tantric way
> Should firstly acquire the essential empowerments.

Also it is said in chapter two of *The Diamond Rosary Tantra* (Skt. *Vajramala tantra*),

> Empowerment is of primary importance;
> All the attainments rest constantly within it.
> I will explain the significance of empowerment;
> You should listen well to what is said.
>
> If in the beginning the trainees
> Are given the complete empowerments,
> They become complete vessels at that time
> For practicing the completion stage yogas.
>
> However, if while lacking the tantric empowerments
> A practitioner learns the meaning of tantra,

> Both guru and disciple equally
> Will end up in the hells.

As clearly stated in the above scriptures, becoming an appropriate vessel for listening to or meditating upon the Secret Path relies upon receiving the according empowerments. Therefore the empowerments are called "the root of all siddhis." Without the empowerments it is impossible to achieve any of the special siddhis, no matter how much teaching is understood or practice undertaken.

Not only is there the fault that profound accomplishment is impossible without first having received the empowerments, in addition, even if one does gain some small siddhi, nonetheless both master and disciple will fall into the hell realms.

On the topic of the empowerments *The Root Tantra of Chakrasamvara* (Skt. *Chakrasamvara mula tantra*) states,

> If a mantra practitioner, without having been introduced into
>   the mandala,
> Attempts to practice the tantric yogas,
> It will be like punching at the empty sky,
> Or like drinking the water of a mirage.

Thus as a preliminary to tantric practice one should be introduced into the mandala, should observe the mandala, and should be given the empowerments, such as the water initiation, crown initiation, and so forth.[14]

Otherwise, if one has the basis of having previously received empowerment into some other mandala [than the one appropriate to the specific practice being undertaken], then it is acceptable to receive only selected portions of the related empowerment, or to receive a blessing initiation.[15] However, if you have not previously received a complete empowerment, then a simple blessing initiation will not adequately serve the purpose. This is stated in the original tantric scriptures; it was taught by the Indian panditas and mahasiddhas; and it is the advice of the Tibetan lineage lamas.

Moreover, it is best if here the empowerment is into a mandala from either the Hevajra or Chakrasamvara cycles. These two have a special connection [with the Six Yogas system].[16]

Why it is necessary to observe the tantric precepts

At the time of receiving tantric empowerment one pledges to cultivate the precepts and commitments of tantric practice. This is done in the presence of the initiation master, as well as [the visualized assembly] of gurus, buddhas and bodhisattvas. One should observe these guidelines, and practice accordingly. As is said in *The Root Tantra of Chakrasamvara*,

> The practitioner engaged in intense tantric training
> Should constantly maintain the tantric precepts.
> If the precepts become weakened,
> No siddhi is achieved from initiation into the mandala.

Also, *The Tantra of Interpenetrating Union* (Skt. *Shri samayoga tantra*) states,

> Not to have been introduced into the mandala,
> To ignore the tantric precepts,
> And not to have understood the essence of secrets:
> To practice on that basis produces no attainment.

As said above, no matter how long or how intensely one practices the tantric yogas, the desired effects will not arise if one has not first received the appropriate empowerments into the mandala; or if one abandons the tantric precepts that are to be maintained; or if one does not thoroughly understand the key points in the two stages of tantric practice.

Those who claim to be practitioners of highest yoga tantra, yet do not even know the number of root and branch precepts, will gain no results. It is important to gain a clear understanding of the root and branch precepts, and to guard them well.[17]

The preliminaries emphasized in this Naropa system

The supreme preliminary preparation involves training the mind in the basic practices [as explained earlier], receiving the pure tantric empowerments, and then correctly guarding the root and branch tantric precepts. One should be clear on this.

In general, the exclusively tantric preliminaries as found in most traditions include the practices of guru yoga, the Vajrasattva mantra recitation and meditation, the offering of the mandala, and so forth.

However, in the teachings of the lineage masters of the Six Yogas tradition, two of the above are separately explained: the meditation and mantra recitation of Vajrasattva, undertaken in order to purify the mind of negative karmic seeds and obscurations; and the devotional meditations of guru yoga, undertaken in order to establish strong waves of blessing power on the mind.

[*Translator's note:* I have placed Tsongkhapa's treatment of the Vajrasattva meditation in Appendix I and his treatment of the Guru

Yoga meditation in Appendix II. Readers who want to follow the text of *A Book of Three Inspirations* in its original order can do so by turning here to those appendices. However, I recommend that the non-specialist first work through Tsongkhapa's treatment of the Six Yogas themselves, and then read these appendices.][18]

Having established the preliminaries, how to train in the actual tantric meditations

This involves two subjects: the meditations of the generation stage yogas; and the meditations of the completion stage yogas.

THE MEDITATIONS OF THE GENERATION STAGE YOGAS

As for the first of these, the meditations on the generation stage yogas, some Tibetan traditions propound the erroneous view that the generation stage yogas are only necessary for the accomplishment of the worldly siddhis [such as meditative concentration, paranormal psychic abilities, magical powers, etc.], and are not needed for accomplishing the supreme siddhi [i.e., the experience of enlightenment wisdom].

However, in three of the [four] principal lineages coming from Lama Marpa—the Mey lineage (Tib. *Mes lugs*), the Tsur lineage (Tib. *mTshur lugs*), and the Ngok lineage (Tib. *rNgog lugs*)—the instruction of the generation stage yogas was always given before the instruction of the completion stage yogas.[19]

This was also the case with [the fourth principal lineage from Marpa, that of] the Venerable Milarepa. As he himself put it,

> In order to train the mind in skillful perception
> Of the events that occur in the bardo between birth and death,
> One should apply oneself to both the generation and completion stage yogas.

Many other great masters of the past have similarly taught the necessity for meditating upon both the generation and completion stage yogas, pointing out that not to become proficient in the generation stage before entering into the completion stage yogas contradicts the advice of both the original tantric scriptures [taught by Buddha] and the later authoritative Indian treatises. It also contradicts this tradition [i.e., the legacy of the Six Yogas of Naropa]. Therefore one should definitely practice the generation stage yogas before entering into the completion stage practices.[20] *The Hevajra Tantra* states,

> Abiding equally in the two stages of tantric practice
> Is the Dharma taught by Buddha Vajradhara.

And also,

> The practitioner meditates upon [the visualized] fabrication
>   [i.e., the generation stage yogas].
> By meditating upon the dream-like quality of the fabrication,
> The fabrication goes beyond fabrication.

The great [Indian] master Nagarjuna himself said,

> Firstly establish yourself well in the generation stage yogas
> And then aspire to the completion stage yogas.
> This is the method taught by the Buddha.
> These [two yogas] are like the steps of a ladder.

Thus all the authoritative tantric scriptures teach that one should meditate upon the generation stage before taking up the completion stage yogas. The main purpose of the actual generation stage yogas is to prepare and ripen the mindstream for the realizations and experiences that are induced through the completion stage yogas.[21]

Moreover, when one achieves a firm samadhi [i.e., meditative power] on the generation stage [through meditation upon a complete mandala], then one can use a yoga system from [a simpler] mandala of a single pair of male and female deities for the completion stage training, and there will be fewer dangers. However, doing so from the beginning [i.e., using a simplified mandala from the beginning] is not the intent of the tantric treatises.

Just how should one pursue meditation on the generation stage yogas?

According to the authoritative teachers and lineage masters of the tradition, the foundation of the path [of the Six Yogas of Naropa] is the practice of the inner heat yoga. In turn, the principal source of this teaching is the Hevajra Tantra. Therefore [the generation stage may be performed on the basis of] the mandalas of any of the four families of Hevajra.[22]

However, many of the previous masters who treasured this oral tradition [of the Six Yogas] accomplished the generation stage yogas in reliance upon the Heruka Chakrasamvara mandala meditations [instead of the Hevajra mandala].

For example, Gampopa relied upon the lineage of Maryul Loden, the disciple of Zangkar. This was known as "the Chakrasamvara lineage of Zangkar."

Also, the glorious Pakmo Drupa relied upon the Chakrasamvara transmission from Lochung (Tib. *Lo chung nas brgyud pa*; lit., "the lineage from the Junior Translator"), known as the Mar lineage.

Moreover, the Dharma master Chojey Drikungpa relied upon the Chakrasamvara tradition of Lama Chokro, which is the lineage from Mardo (Tib. *Mar do'i lugs*).[23]

All three of the above Chakrasamvara lineages are based upon the sixty-two deity mandala of Heruka Chakrasamvara known as the tradition of [the Indian mahasiddha] Luipada.

Thus there are these two mandalas [Hevajra and Heruka Chakrasamvara, that have been used by great lineage masters of the past]. The teaching on *tummo*, the inner heat yoga, is common to both of them. Thus either mandala practice is appropriate [as the basis of the generation stage yoga to be used as the preparation for the completion stage yogas]. Meditation upon the mandala of a solitary male or female deity will not have the same power of effectively ripening the mindstream as will meditating upon the generation stage yogas associated with a complete mandala. The mandala should be at least as complete as that of the five-deity Heruka Chakrasamvara mandala of the Ghantapada tradition (Tib. *Dril bu zhabs kyi lha lnga*).[24]

Adopting one of the above mandalas as the basis, one engages in the practice in four daily yogic sessions.

The manner of inducing the desired experiences from the generation stage yogas is to begin by cultivating a panoramic meditative visualization free from mental wanderings. If the principal mandala deity has many faces and arms, in the beginning one should relax one's focus upon the details and concentrate instead on the main face and main two arms, fixing one's attention upon the visualization of them.

Here there are two aspects to the training: radiant appearance and tantric pride.

One cultivates the first of these by moving one's awareness from the top downward, and then from the feet upward, flowing through the visualized form, and thus cultivating a rough image of the mandala deity and its attributes. Eventually one is able to sense the image as a whole. One holds the image firmly yet gently, concentrating upon it single-pointedly. In the beginning the image will not come clearly, and other images will force it to fade. One simply returns the mind to the visualization when one notices this happening. If the image becomes unclear, rejuvenate the visualization and continue meditating. One pursues the training in this way, and the radiant presence of the image gradually increases.

Thus one cultivates the radiant presence of the visualized image. Thought-flows other than the desired one gradually cease to arise, and the visualization becomes more radiantly present and vivid than a physical form seen by the eye. One must place the mind on that radiant presence [of the visualized mandala], without falling prey to either of the two obstacles, torpor and agitation, during the session.

If in this way one succeeds in generating the visualization of the simple two-armed form of the mandala deity, one goes on to cultivate the visualization of the other arms, the ornaments, and so forth, until the visualized image of the complete form of the mandala deity has been mastered, using the method [of sweeping and focusing] as before. Then one goes on to cultivate the visualization of the consort, and eventually the other mandala deities.

One should continue like that until finally one arrives at a stage wherein the entire host of supported mandala deities and the supporting mandala, coarse and subtle, can be generated in the mind in a single moment, and wherein one can maintain that visualization single-pointedly for a protracted period of time.[25]

As for the training in the methods of cultivating divine pride, the point here is to generate the strong thought that one is the very mandala deity, and to rest the mind single-pointedly in that conviction. Whenever this tantric self-awareness begins to wane, rejuvenate the pride of being the mandala deity as before, and place the mind there.

In the beginning this meditation is in the nature of a mental fabrication. Eventually it becomes stable, and one achieves a sense of divine tantric pride that spontaneously pervades the conscious mind.

The trainings should also be cultivated in the periods between formal meditation sittings.

From the very beginning of the generation stage yogas these two aspects of practice—divine pride and the radiant appearance of the mandala—should be cultivated as complementary. When our meditation on the supported mandala deities and supporting mandala achieves maturity, the mere mindfulness of the radiantly present image will give rise to a wonderful sense of being in which the ordinary appearances of things do not arise. Thus the technique has the power to purify from within the mind the mundane presence of the conventional world. Similarly, if one can generate a strong sense of unfeigned divine pride as explained earlier, this will have the power to purify from within the mind the habit of apprehending things as mundane.

One arises from formal meditation and goes about daily activities, seeing the manifestations of the world and living beings as mandala and tantric deities. This is the samadhi that transforms the world and its living beings into a most extraordinary vision. This is what is meant by the expression, "The generation stage yogas purify mundane appearance and apprehension." As is said in *The Arising of Samvara Tantra* (Skt. *Samvarodaya tantra*),

> The three realms of the world
> Are by nature the mandala's inconceivable mansion;
> And all the living beings of the world
> Are by nature mandala deities.

Also [the Indian mahasiddha] Aryadeva said, "If you understand this world and its inhabitants as mandala and deities, then how can you, O mind, ever become confused?"

This principle applies equally to both stages of tantric practice [generation and completion]. On [both stages in] Vajrayana practice, all that appears is brought into the circle of the mandala; all experiences are taken as manifestations of great ecstasy; and all thoughts are sealed as being unborn and uncreated.

This is present throughout the generation stage. And although on the generation stage there is not the presence of the actual great ecstasy that is aroused on the completion stage by means of bringing the vital energies into the central channel, or *avadhuti*, one should appreciate that when the practitioner achieves stability in the vision of himself or herself as the male and female deities in sexual union, experiencing the visualization as though it were real, at that point method and wisdom enter into a balanced union. Subsequent to that the mantric syllable "PEH" (Skt. *PHAT*) is enounced [in the daily *sadhana*, or liturgical meditation] in order to prevent the bodhimind substance from exiting the body, and various levels of great ecstasy occur. This is the ecstasy of the generation stage.

These are the principal means by which the practice of the generation stage ripens the mind for the completion stage yogas.

THE MEDITATIONS OF THE COMPLETION STAGE YOGAS

This will be explained under three headings: the explanation of the nature of the basis; the explanation of the stages of traversing the path; and the manner of actualizing the results.

The nature of the basis

This involves two subjects: the nature of the mind; and the nature of the body.

To convey a sense of the deeper nature of the subject of meditation, the first of these is taught. To convey a sense of the energy centers of the body that will be meditated upon, the second is taught.[26]

The nature of the mind

Here the ultimate nature of the mind is taught first. The approach is described in *The Hevajra Tantra in Two Sections* (Skt. *Hevajra tantra nama*), wherein we read,

> By nature there is no form, no perceiver,
> No sound, and no hearer of sound,
> No aromas, and no perceivers of aromas,
> No taste, and no experiencer of taste,
> No physical sensations, and no experiencer of them,
> No mind, and no mental events.

Elsewhere the same text states,

> The sensory powers, the objects of the senses,
> And likewise the sensory consciousnesses
> Are known to be the yoginis [of the mandala].
> All eighteen *dhatus* of experience are understood in this way.

> By nature from the very beginning they are uncreated,
> And likewise are not false and not true;
> All phenomena are like the moon reflected in water.
> The yoginis appreciate things in this way.

Here the five sensory realms—form, sound, scents, tastes and sensations—and also the five sensory powers that experience these—from the perceiver of form, etc., to the experiencer of sensations—from the eye power to the body power—all are classified as sensory powers. In terms of the five psychophysical aggregates (Skt. *skandha*), all the above belong to the skandha of form. In the context of the gateways of experience (Skt. *ayatana*), they are known as the ten gateways of form. All of these are without any inherent, real existence.

"Mind" includes the skandha of awareness and the ayatana of consciousness. "Mental events" includes [the skandhas of] feelings, distinguishing awareness and mentative patterns.

Using these as examples, the gateway of the phenomena which are objects of experience of the mind are shown to be non-truly existent.

Similarly, in the above verse, we see the words "no perceiver." This points to the perceiver of form, hearer of sounds, and so forth. These lead to the subject of the "person," the sense of "I." Thus this too is empty of true existence.

In brief, all that exists, both persons and phenomena, are shown to be selflessness without an inherently real nature.

As for the manner in which they lack self-nature, this is introduced by the words [in the above verse, wherein it is said] "by nature... not...." All phenomena, including persons, forms and so forth, are without a nature that is inherently real.

This is the interpretation given by [the Indian] mahasiddha Padma in his commentary on the subject. It has the same sense as the scriptural passages that speak of "by nature non-existent" and "without self-characteristics." Other similar expressions are "without self-nature," and "without true essence."

"By nature... uncreated" implies that the situation is not such that at some point in the past the phenomena were without this nature of emptiness of true existence, and that through reason and scriptural sayings they came to have an emptiness nature. From primordial time all things have lacked true existence. A verse by Lama Marpa states,

> I travelled east to the banks of the Ganges River
> And there, through the kindness of Guru Maitripa,
> Realized the uncreated nature of phenomena.
> I seized with my bare hands the emptiness nature of my mind,
> Beheld the primordial essence beyond concepts,
> Directly encountered the mother of the three kayas,
> And severed the net of my confusion.

Thus Lama Marpa himself states that he acquired his realization of the mahamudra doctrine principally from his training with the [Indian] mahasiddha Maitripa.[27]

A treatise by that master [i.e., Maitripa], entitled *Ten Reflections on Simple Suchness* (Skt. *Tattva dashaka*), [states,] "If you wish to experience the quintessential nature of being [i.e., voidness], be aware that it is not 'with characteristics' and not 'without characteristics'."

The meaning here is that if one wishes to understand the quintessential nature of being, then one should not take the approach to emptiness taught by the [Indian Buddhist] schools that speak of [emptiness] "with characteristics" and "without characteristics."

The mahasiddha Maitripa's direct disciple, the pandit Sahajavajra, explains that in the scriptures of the Shravakas we see a discussion of "emptiness with characteristics," as is popular with the Sautrantika school of [Indian Buddhist] thought; and "emptiness without characteristics," as is popular with the Vaibhashika school. Moreover, he continues, in the [Mahayana schools such as] the Vijnanavadin, we see a discussion of emptiness having "true and false characteristics," and in the Yogachara Madhyamaka school, the doctrine of "conventionally true characteristics and conventionally false characteristics."

The same text continues,

> One should rely upon the approach to emptiness elucidated by the great Madhyamaka masters Arya Nagarjuna, Aryadeva, Chandrakirti, and so forth, who teach that the interdependent, co-existent nature of phenomena points to the suchness of being. We should adopt the guidelines set forth by these three masters.

Here Acharya Nagarjuna and Aryadeva are the early forefathers of the Madhyamaka school [of Indian Buddhism]. Many later Indian masters followed their tradition. They had many different followers [over the centuries], who explained the Madhyamaka in various ways. The master Maitripa is among them, and is said to be a follower of Chandrakirti. [Maitripa's] *Ten Reflections on Simple Suchness* states,

> To put it plainly, most of these gurus are merely
> Unadorned, mediocre teachers of the Middle View.

What he means is that most teachers are not adorned with the oral tradition teachings from Chandrakirti. They are but mediocre proponents of the Middle View, and rely upon mediocre lineages of the emptiness doctrine. In this tradition Chandrakirti represents the most quintessential expression of the emptiness doctrine [coming from Nagarjuna and Aryadeva]. One should follow the approach [to emptiness] outlined by him.

The meaning of the expression "not true and not false" is explained in [Nagarjuna's treatise] *Sixty Stanzas on the Nature of Emptiness* (Skt. *Yukti shashtika*),

> All the various objects of experience
> Are like the moon reflected in water—
> Neither really true nor really false.
> Those appreciating this do not lose the view.

One should understand the emptiness doctrine in the context of this simile. The wise perceive that all things—persons and phenomena—arise in reliance upon their own causes and conditions, and that based on this process we impute mental labels upon things. The phenomena themselves have no true or inherent existence from their own side. They have no self-nature whatsoever.

Were persons or phenomena to have a self-presence, there would be no need for them to rely upon causes and conditions. Therefore one can be certain that even the smallest speck of matter has no true, inherent existence from its own side.

Although all things lack even the smallest speck of true existence, nonetheless conventionally the laws of causes and conditions operate through them, and conventionally all the phenomena in samsara and nirvana seem to exist, arising in the same manner as do illusions, dreams and a reflected image.

However, phenomena are not false in the sense that the saying "A horn on a rabbit's head exists" is false. Nor is it a matter of a superficial, conventional distortion alone, like the rope seen in the dark that is mistaken for a snake.

The view of emptiness to be understood is the reality of how all things lack even the smallest particle of true, inherent existence.

Otherwise, if one does not arrive at this meditative understanding, then the method will not bring even liberation from cyclic existence, let alone produce the state of complete enlightenment.

Therefore *The Vajra Tent Tantra* (Skt. *Vajra panjara*) states,

> In order to reverse the habit of grasping at an I,
> The buddhas have taught the doctrine of emptiness.

The meaning is that in order to reverse the trend of apprehending a self in persons and phenomena, the buddhas have taught that one must ascertain the meaning of emptiness.

As the great masters of the past have pointed out, all phenomena, which ultimately are only names and mental labels, nonetheless on the conventional level function validly, albeit in the nature of a distortion, an illusion, and a dream. Not to appreciate this [valid conventional nature of things] is a great mistake, and is an unhealthy philosophical excess. If one takes the theory of emptiness too far, one easily falls over the precipice of nihilism. Thus it is crucial to appreciate how, on the conventional level, things operate according to the principles of illusion-like interdependent arising.[28]

That one should understand the nature of the two levels of truth—ultimate and conventional—in this way was expressed as follows by Milarepa, that great yogi and master of this path, in the following song:

> For those of weaker minds the omniscient Buddha taught,
> To accord with the predispositions of those to be trained,
> That the objects of knowledge have real existence;
> But from the perspective of higher truth, nothing
> From a hindering spirit to a buddha has real existence.
>
> There are no meditators, no objects of meditation,
> No spiritual progress, no path with signs,
> No resultant kayas, no wisdom,
> And therefore no nirvana.
>
> Solely by means of names and mental labels
> The stable and moving elements of the three worlds
> Are established; in reality from the very beginning
> They are unproduced, uncreated, baseless, innately unborn.
>
> There is no karma nor ripening effects of actions,
> And therefore even the name "samsara" does not exist.
> This is the sense of the final truth.

Thus from the perspective of the ultimate level of reality it is said that not the smallest particle of anything in samsara or nirvana has even the slightest trace of true existence. However, elsewhere Milarepa said,

> Eh-ma! Yet if there are no living beings, how then
> Can the buddhas of the three times come into being?
> Without a cause, there can be no effect.
>
> From the perspective of conventional reality,
> All things in samsara and nirvana,
> Which the Buddha has accepted as conventionally valid,
> All existents, things, appearances, non-existents,
> All these functional realities, are inseparably

Of one taste with the quintessential nature of emptiness.
There is no self-awareness, and no other-awareness.
All share in the vastness of yuganaddha, the great union.

The wise who realize this truth
No longer see mind, but only wisdom-mind.
They no longer see living beings, only buddhas.
They no longer see phenomena, only the quintessential nature.

Thus from the perspective of ultimate reality even the names of the phenomena in samsara do not exist. Yet conventionally, so that the living beings can traverse the path to buddhahood, the conventional level of reality [such as cause and effect, etc.] is spoken of as existing. However, its status is conventionally established solely on the basis of imputed names and labels. In reality these interdependent manifestations of appearing phenomena are emptiness lacking any inherent existence.

These two levels of truth—the conventional reality of functioning occurrences and the ultimate reality of emptiness—abide always in one taste. The manifest and the emptiness natures are never separable from one another. The ultimate level points to and supports the conventional; and the conventional points to and supports the ultimate.

This manner in which the presence of every phenomenon simultaneously reveals both ultimate and conventional levels of reality is a key point of the masters of this tradition [of the Naropa Six Yogas]. In the process of ascertaining the middle view it advises that we follow the guidelines of the great Madhyamaka treatises.

One should not think that in this tradition [i.e., the Six Yogas transmission] we don't have to speak in terms of the two levels of truth. To do otherwise is to contradict the Buddha's own teachings, as well as the treatises of the early Indian masters. It also contradicts the tradition of the Six Yogas.

To arrive at the correct understanding of "the union of ecstasy and void" one should apply oneself to gaining an understanding of emptiness as outlined above [i.e., one should follow the guidelines as presented by Nagarjuna, Aryadeva and Chandrakirti].

The nature of the body

This introduces the subjects of the "energy channel wheels" (Skt. *chakra*), such as "the chakra of emanation at the navel"; the upper and lower regions of the central energy channel (Skt. *avadhuti*; Tib.

rtsa dbu ma) that are to be stimulated through application of the profound tantric technology; and so forth.[29]

According to the holders of the oral tradition of the Marpa lineage, these tantric yogas are to be practiced during both the sleeping and waking states.

With the first of these [i.e., when working with the sleep state], one should understand the key points of stimulating the chakras at the heart and throat. Then during the waking state one works with the chakras at the navel and crown, the former in connection with the inner heat yoga, and the latter in connection with the yoga of sexual union with a karmamudra. This is because on those occasions the subtle drops (Skt. *bindu*) that support consciousness abide within those four sites. The tradition [of the Six Yogas] speaks in this way.

This subject is also discussed in the system of the Kalachakra Tantra, wherein it is said that the chakras at the forehead and navel are associated with the waking state; the chakras at the throat and secret place are associated with the dream state; the chakras at the heart and jewel are associated with deep sleep; and the chakras at the navel and tip of the secret place are associated with the state of the fourth occasion [i.e., sexual ecstasy]. Thus the presentations of the two systems are similar in this way.

When one enters into sleep, the subtle energies collect into the chakras at the heart and jewel. As long as they remain there, one experiences a deep, dreamless sleep. Should they begin to dissipate from these two chakras and collect into the chakras at the throat and secret place, one will begin to experience dreams. One will continue to dream for as long as the energies remain in these two chakras. When the energies leave these sites and move to the chakras at the forehead and navel one awakens from sleep altogether.

When the bodhimind substance descends from the forehead chakra and comes to the chakras at the navel and tip of the jewel, it induces an experience of transformative bliss as it passes through each of the chakras. This is the experience of the fourth occasion [i.e., ecstasy]. This can be induced by means of training in the tantric yogas, which bring control over the subtle bodily energies. By means of this process of energy control the drop is brought down [from the crown chakra to] the navel chakra, giving rise to the "descending from above" innate bliss; and, for a more profound and complete experience, the drop is brought to the chakra at the tip of the jewel.

The fact that these four chakras are stimulated during the states of sleep and dream does not mean that they are inaccessible during the waking state.

From among the chakras, in this tradition [i.e., the Six Yogas] one begins the practice by working with the "wheel of emanation," which is the chakra at the navel.

Meditating on the individual chakras produces individual effects, and these must be understood in the stream of one's own experience.

The explanation of the stages of traversing the path

This is taught under two headings: the meditations upon the physical exercises, together with the meditation upon the body as an empty shell; and, secondly, after that, the stages of meditating upon the actual path.

The meditations upon the physical exercises, together with the meditation upon the body as empty

According to the oral traditions of some later teachers in the Marpa lineage, at this point in the training one establishes protection through meditation on the syllable *HUM*, in conjunction with the threefold practice of collecting, absorbing and retaining [the vital energies]. [Those later teachers] also establish protection by means of relying upon small wrathful [deities], and by accumulating positive energy through the practice of guru yoga. In their traditions the physical exercises and meditations upon the body as an empty shell are not used.[30]

However, the lineage that passed from Milarepa to Gampopa did not include the former three. It instead advocated the physical exercises and the meditation upon the body as an empty shell. Hence it seems that there are two ways of explaining the Six Yogas of Naropa: the system as taught by the earlier masters; and the system as taught by many later masters. This treatise will follow the former approach.

[The meditations upon the physical exercises]

One begins each session of the physical exercises by chanting the verses of refuge, generating the universal aspiration of the bodhisattva way, and then meditating upon the guru as seated upon a lotus above one's head, together with offering verses of supplication for blessings. One does these until one's mindstream is blended with them. One then visualizes oneself as the mandala deity, male and female in sexual union. Every session should be commenced in this way.

Different traditions recommend different numbers of physical exercises, as well as exactly how to do them. Here we will follow the instructions of glorious Pakmo Drupa.

In glorious Pakmo Drupa's manual [on the Six Yogas], entitled *Verses on the Path Technology: A Supplement* (Tib. *Thabs lam tshigs bcad ma'i lhan thabs*), [it is stated]:

> There are six exercises for purifying the body: filling like a vase; circling like a wheel; hooking like a hook; showing the mudra of vajra binding, lifting upward toward the sky, and then pressing downward; straightening like an arrow, and then forcefully releasing the air in the manner of a dog heaving; and, in order to energize the passageways and blood in the body, shaking the head and entire body and flexing the muscles. These are the six.

These are the techniques famed as the "six exercises of Naropa."

As said above, the first is that of filling the body like a vase. One sits on a comfortable cushion, with the legs crossed comfortably. The back is set straight and the two hands placed on the knees.

One draws in air through the right nostril, gazes to the left, and then releases it through the left, exhaling slowly and gently until no more remains [in the lungs]. One then draws in air through the left nostril, gazes to the right, and gently releases it via the other nostril. Next one draws in the air through both nostrils, gazes straight ahead, and releases it slowly through both.

One repeats this cycle of three breaths two more times, thus making nine breaths. In this way the breath is purified. Throughout the process no air is to be allowed to pass through the mouth on either inhalation or exhalation.

One now sits with the body straight and erect, and the hands formed into fists with the thumbs inside. One breathes in slowly and deeply, while pulling the air down to below the navel. One then swallows some saliva without making a sound, pressing down [the swallowed liquid] with the abdomen to a point just below the navel chakra. Also, one pulls up from below [with the muscles of the pelvic floor], retaining the air inside in this way. With awareness poised at the center of the navel chakra, one holds the breath for as long as one can. In this way the body is filled [with air] like a full vase.

As all the subsequent physical exercises are performed in conjunction with this breathing technique, it is only counted as a separate exercise for the sake of convenience.

When one can no longer hold the air inside, one releases it slowly through the nostrils, not allowing any to escape through the mouth. Exhalation should always be done in this way, without exception.

The second exercise is that of circling like a wheel. Begin by sitting in the vajra posture. Then hold the big toe of the right foot with the right hand, and the big toe of the left foot with the left hand. One straightens the spine, and then rolls the upper waist and stomach clockwise three times. One then rolls them counterclockwise three times. Next one stretches the upper body from the left to the right, and then from the right to the left. Finally one snaps the solar plexus from the front toward the back, and then from the back toward the front.

For the third exercise, that of hooking like a hook, one forms the hands into vajra fists and then, with muscles tensed, stretches them outward, from the heart to directly in front of the chest. One then stretches the two arms to the left, and slowly but with muscles tensed slides the right hand back to the right shoulder. One next brings the left hand to the heart, and snaps the left elbow into the rib cage. This is repeated three times. Now, just as was done to the left above, one does the same in reverse. One makes the vajra fist mudra, beginning with the two hands at the heart and then extending them straight outward slowly but with tensed muscles. One now stretches them to the right, hooks them as before [except in reverse], bringing the left hand to the left shoulder, the right hand to the heart, and snapping the right elbow into the rib cage.

The fourth exercise is that of showing the mudra of vajra binding, lifting upward toward the sky, and then pressing downward. Plant the knees flat [on the floor], straighten the body, and then, with the fingers of both hands outstretched upward like metal hooks, one lifts upward slowly but with great intensity to above the crown. One then reverses the hands [to have the hooked fingers pointing downward], and brings them down slowly but with intensity.

Fifthly is the exercise of making the body straight as an arrow and then [expelling the air] with the sound of a dog heaving. Kneel on the floor, straighten the body, place the hands on the floor, and put your head in between [the hands]. Slowly yet with intensity raise the head and straighten the body. Then bring the head back down to between the two hands [while keeping the arms straight], and forcefully expel all air from the lungs, uttering the sound "hah," like a dog heaving. Then stand up and shake the feet three times each.

The sixth exercise is that of shaking the head and body, and flexing the joints. One pulls on the fingers of the two hands [in order to pop the joints], and then shakes the head and body all over. Finally, massage the two hands, as though washing them.

While practicing these physical exercises one should retain the breath and control the vital energies. The movements should be slow yet intense. The time for practice is before eating [i.e., when the stomach is empty], or some time after having eaten, when the stomach has relaxed from the food. Do them until the body becomes totally flexible.

[The meditations on the body as an empty shell]

In the meditations on the body as an empty shell (Tib. *stong ra*), one commences as before with the practice of visualizing oneself as the mandala deity. The special application here is to concentrate on the body, from the tip of the head to the soles of the feet, as being utterly empty of material substance, like an empty transparent balloon filled with light. Place the mind firmly and clearly on this image.

This meditation [on the body as empty, or immaterial] and the physical exercises should be practiced in conjunction with one another.

Here the body is to be envisioned as being entirely without substance, appearing in the mind like a rainbow in the sky. Although this practice cannot transform the body into that nature, nonetheless it is very beneficial to visualize it in this way and to keep the mind on that image. One immediate benefit is that the forceful meditations for controlling the vital energies and opening the subtle channels will not cause pain from the changing energy flows or from the opening of the channels. And even if some pain does occur, these meditations on the empty-shell body will mitigate it. These are the special effects of this meditation. The physical exercises have similar beneficial effects.

There are many different versions of this meditation on the process of the empty-shell body. There are also many unauthentic versions of the practice. What is explained above is in accordance with the guidelines given by the glorious Pakmo Drupa and may therefore be regarded as sufficient.

These two techniques—the physical exercises, and the empty-shell body—are not mentioned in the principal tantric texts translated from

Sanskrit into Tibetan. However, they are found in the writings of the oral traditions as transmitted by the gurus of old.

When we meditate on the chakras, it is sometimes difficult solely by means of gentle preparatory methods to induce a state of samadhi having the ability to control the vital energies and to open the energy channels. When these more forceful preliminaries are done, there is less chance of undesirable side-effects occurring.

The stages of meditating upon the actual path

This will be explained under two headings: the manner of structuring the path; and the stages of being guided on the path.

The manner of structuring the path

There are many ways of structuring this system of tantric yoga, the most common being into two, three, four, six and ten branches.[31]

Here Gampopa, classifying it in accordance with the capacities of the trainees, presented it in three ways: for those who could accomplish enlightenment in this lifetime; for those who could accomplish it in the bardo, which follows the moment of death; and for those who could accomplish it over a period of a stream of lifetimes.

Elsewhere, when Gampopa classified it in accordance with the nature of the path to be meditated upon, he gives a twofold breakdown: the general completion stage yogas, the power of which leads one across the path; and the methods and activities of the enhancement techniques. As for the second of these, they do not appear in the traditions of those lineages of the Naropa system that depend principally upon the oral instruction transmissions. Almost no oral instruction tradition contains them. However, they can be found in the traditions of the explanatory lineages coming from Lama Marpa.[32]

Lama Marpa himself said,

> At the feet of the gatekeeper, the mighty Pandita Naropa,
> I listened to the profound tantric teachings of the Hevajra
>   system.
> There I received the precepts on blending, transference and
>   union.
> In particular, I received the instructions
> On inner heat yoga and the practice of karmamudra yoga,
> And was introduced to the key points of the whispered
>   tradition.

Thus Marpa in general was introduced to the secret whispered tradition[33] on the threefold practice of blending, transference and union. In particular, by relying on the Hevajra Tantra teachings he learned the methods of inducing the four blisses through both the inner practice of heat yoga and the outer practice of karmamudra yoga. Thus he mainly mastered these two—the inner heat doctrine and karmamudra—based principally on the Hevajra Root Tantra.

Elsewhere Lama Marpa said,

> In the west, in the town of Tulakshetra,
> I bowed at the feet of the glorious Jnanagarbha
> And listened to the Guhyasamaja Tantra, a male tantric system.
> There I received the instructions on the illusory body and clear
>   light
> And trained in the essence of the five stages of the path.

As Marpa himself states here, on the one side he relied upon the transmission known as "the four exalted instructions" from the lineage of Naropa;[34] and also he relied upon the instructions of the "Five Stages" tradition of the Guhyasamaja Tantra. This latter he received in separate transmissions from both Jnanagarbha and Naropa, and thus the traditions of the illusory body yoga and clear light yoga [in his lineage] mainly derive from the Guhyasamaja Tantra's "Five Stages" technology.[35]

As for the yogic techniques of consciousness transference and "forceful projection," it seems that he mainly assimilated these from *The Four Seats Tantra* (Skt. *Shri chaturpitha tantra*).

The list of the Six Yogas is as follows: inner heat; illusory body; clear light; consciousness transference; forceful projection; and the bardo yoga.

Here dream yoga and bardo yoga are both branches of the illusory body yoga. Moreover, "the clear-light-of-sleep yoga" is also subsumed under the instruction of the illusory body.

The instructions on consciousness transference and on forceful projection are usually explained together, for the sake of convenience.

Jetsun Milarepa described the oral transmission that he had received from Marpa as follows:

> The tradition of Marpa of the Southern Hills has six instructions: the generation stage yogas; inner heat; karmamudra; introduction to the essence of the view of the ultimate nature of being; the indicative clear light of the path; and the indicative illusory nature, together with dream yoga. This is the heart-essence of

> Marpa's teachings. There is no higher precept for introducing the trainee to the essence of the whispered teachings. There is no more precious instruction than this, the heart of that yogi's thought. No teaching is more practical.

Of these six, all but the first belong to the completion stage techniques.

The traditions of the holders of the explanatory transmissions of the tantras coming from Lama Marpa are in harmony with what is said here [by Milarepa]. Therefore those who claim to hold lineages [coming from Lama Marpa] more profound than the Six Yogas of Naropa are only fooling themselves.

In general, all systems of highest yoga tantra's completion stage involve the preliminary process of controlling the vital energies flowing through the two side channels, *rasana* and *lalana*, and redirecting them into the central channel, *avadhuti*. This is indispensable.[36]

There are numerous means for accomplishing this, based on the traditions of the Indian mahasiddhas, who drew from the various tantric systems. In this tradition [i.e., the Six Yogas of Naropa] the main technique is to arouse the inner heat at the navel chakra, the "wheel of emanation," and then through controlling the life energies by means of the *AH*-stroke mantric syllable [lit., "the short *AH*], to draw the subtle life-sustaining energies into the central channel. When these energies enter the central channel the four blisses are induced, and one cultivates meditation on the basis of these in such a way as to give rise to the innate wisdom of mahamudra.

Otherwise, if one does not rely upon a profound path of this nature [i.e., in which the basis of the meditation is not the innate ecstasy conjoined with wisdom awareness], but instead engages a samadhi that merely maintains a state of non-conceptual absorption for a prolonged period of time, no great signs of progress will be produced. Firm concentration placed in a state of pleasant, clear non-conceptuality is a practice common to both the Hinayana and Mahayana; and, within the Mahayana, it is common to both the Paramitayana and Mantrayana. It is important not to confuse the two types of samadhi.

Thus, when Milarepa and Gampopa met for the first time and Gampopa commented that he could sit in meditative concentration for many days at a time without distraction, Milarepa replied to him, "You cannot get oil by crushing sand. The practice of samadhi is not sufficient in and of itself. You should learn my system of inner heat yoga, which redirects the subtle life-sustaining energies into the *AH*-stroke mantric syllable." One should understand this point well.

In this tradition the expression "the inner heat, the foundation," is well known. This is because in the completion stage yogas one uses the inner heat technology from the very beginning in order to collect the subtle life-sustaining energies into the central channel, and thereby arouse the innate great ecstasy. This is the actual basis upon which all practices rely, and upon which all later completion stage yogas are founded. The inner heat doctrine establishes this basis.

The practice of the inner heat doctrine entails directing the life-sustaining energies into the central channel. Here the energies enter, abide, and are dissolved. When one trains well in this technique, the strength of the experience has the power to give control over loss of the bodhimind substance [i.e., the sexual drops]. Then, based on this power, one can rely upon a karmamudra as a conducive condition to arouse the four blisses. On this foundation, innate ecstasy is aroused.

Arousing this innate ecstasy is the purpose of the practices of the inner heat yoga and karmamudra yoga.

One unites the innate ecstasy with [meditation upon] emptiness, and during the waking state applies oneself to the illusory body doctrine. Based on the experience of the illusory body practice one can engage in the clear light technology.

Then when asleep at night one can cultivate awareness of the illusory nature of dreams. To do so effectively one must first master the yoga of retaining the clear light of sleep [i.e., the clear light that arises at the moment of falling asleep], and then enter into the dream state from that perspective. Since the power to retain the clear light of sleep is accomplished by means of gaining control over the vital energies, one must, during the time of waking practice, master this control and cultivate the ability to direct the energies into the central channel. Thus the foundation of both practices [sleep and dream yogas] is the inner heat doctrine.

When one has progressed in the dream yogas, only then can one effectively work with the bardo yogas. Again here [with the bardo yogas] the foundation is the power achieved through the inner heat.

All three of the above yogas [i.e., sleep, dream and bardo] are subsumed under the illusory body yoga.

As for the yogas of special consciousness transference and forceful projection, as a preliminary to them one must cultivate the ability to draw the life-sustaining energies into the central channel. Therefore in these two the inner heat yoga again is the foundation.

If one understands these principles of the system well, then the manner in which the Six Yogas are structured is not important. One should simply adopt the arrangement that feels most comfortable.

The stages of being guided on the path

This will be explained under two headings: the essence of the basic principles in the guidelines of the path; and the methods and activities for enhancing the path.

The essence of the basic principles in the guidelines of the path

The first of these is explained under two headings: the essence of the actual path; and the branches of that path, which include the practices of consciousness transference and forceful projection.

The essence of the actual path

The first of these also has two phases: arousing the four blisses by means of drawing the vital energies into the central channel; and, having accomplished that, the meditations on the illusory body and clear light yogas.

Arousing the four blisses by means of drawing the vital energies into the central channel

Again, the first of these is accomplished by means of assembling two conditions: the inner condition of the meditations on the inner heat yoga; and the external condition of relying upon a karmamudra.

The inner condition of meditations on the inner heat doctrine

Here there are two stages to the practice: meditating upon the inner heat yoga in order to draw the vital energies into the central channel; and, having brought in the energies, the methods of arousing the four blisses.

Meditating upon the inner heat in order to draw the vital energies into the central channel

The first stage is taught under two headings: how to meditate on the inner heat yoga; and by having meditated in this way, how to cause the vital energies to enter, abide and dissolve within the central channel.

How to meditate on the inner heat yoga

Here there are three principal steps in the training: meditating by means of visualizing the channels; meditating by means of visualizing mantric syllables; and meditating by means of engaging the vase breathing technique.

Meditating by means of visualizing the channels

In the first of these one begins by visualizing one's root guru in the space in front, together with the gurus in the line of transmission, surrounded by the host of dakas and dakinis. One symbolically offers them all things without grasping at any, and then follows this with prayers for blessings and realization, making supplication that one's energies may be joyous and energy channels subtle, so that the special realizations of ecstasy and [the wisdom of] emptiness may be easily induced.

One reflects, "For the benefit of living beings as vast in number as the measure of the sky I will achieve the state of a Buddha Vajradhara. For this purpose I now take up the practice of *chandali*, the inner heat yoga." Meditate like this until your stream of being is infused with the bodhimind, the bodhisattva aspiration.

Visualizing yourself as the mandala deity, sit on your meditation seat, put on your meditation belt, cross the legs, and set the backbone erect. The neck is bent slightly forward, and the eyes cast downward at the angle of the nose. The tongue is held gently against the upper palate, and the teeth and lips set in their natural [closed] position. The body and mind are postured alertly, with the chest somewhat extended, and the hands in the meditation posture, placed just under the navel.

One now visualizes the three energy channels. Firstly the central channel, *avadhuti*, is envisioned. It begins at a point four fingerwidths below the navel at the center of the body just in front of the spinal column. To its right is the channel known as *rasana*, and to its left is *lalana*. These channels proceed up the body to the head, like pillars supporting the four chakras.

One imagines that the lower tips of the side channels curve up into the base of the central channel. This is done in order to draw the vital energies into the central channel. Not understanding this purpose, some teachers have said that the three channels just come to an end and stop at a distance four fingerwidths below the navel. Others have said that the two side channels just stop there [at the navel].

[One visualizes the channels in this way for the purpose of meditation. But in fact] the channels continue on down, eventually coming to the tip of the jewel. Above, the central channel comes to the point between the eyebrows, and the two side channels come to the inner passages of the two nostrils.

At the sites of the four chakras, the two side channels, rasana and lalana, wrap around the central channel, forming knots. Otherwise they [all three] run straight [up and down the body].

As for the size of the channels, this varies at times of meditating and not meditating. There is no certain, fixed size.

Moreover, as for the colors of the channels, *A Harvest of Oral Tradition Teachings* (Skt. *Amnaya manjari*) quotes *The Mystic Kiss Tantra* (Skt. *Chaturyogini samputa tantra*) as stating that during the meditation for arousing the inner heat, the central channel should be seen as having the color of the flame produced by burning sesame seed oil. Prior to that point in the training, however, the right channel should be seen as being red, the left white, and the central channel bluish.

Now one visualizes the four chakras. Firstly at the navel is the chakra called "the wheel of emanation." Its shape is somewhat triangular, like the [Sanskrit] syllable *EH*, and it has sixty-four petals. They are red in color, and stretch upward. Meditate upon it in this way. Here the arrangement of the petals is only roughly described. Details are not mentioned; but this is enough.

At the heart is the chakra known as "the wheel of truth." Its shape is somewhat circular, like the [Sanskrit syllable] *BAM*, and it has eight petals, white in color, extending downward.

At the throat is the chakra known as "the wheel of enjoyment," also somewhat circular in shape, like the syllable *BAM*. It has sixteen petals, red in color, reaching upward.

At the crown is the chakra "the wheel of great ecstasy." It also is somewhat triangular, like the syllable *EH*, and has thirty-two petals, is multicolored, and its petals extend downward.

The meditation should hold each of the [two] pairs of chakras within an according embrace of method and wisdom.[37]

When one begins the training of visualizing the three energy channels there are two aspects of the practice to which one should attend, namely, the radiance of the image and the meditative placement. That is to say, one must produce a collection of two factors: the radiant appearance of the envisioned channels; and the firmness of the meditation.

The most important site for the placement of one's awareness at the beginning of practice is the point in the region of the central channel where the three channels join.

Based on this, one proceeds to visualize the four chakras, with their according number of petals, and to fix the mind on them. With persistence in the meditation the chakra petals become increasingly clear [in one's mind], and the mind more firmly placed upon them.

If after considerable effort no clarity is achieved with the chakras, place the mind solely on the image of the three channels. Concentrate especially on the portion above the heart chakra. If still no progress is forthcoming, prolonged application can incur dangerous obstacles. One therefore should relax the application, and place the mind instead on the point where the three channels join [at the lower part of the body].

In this tradition there are two approaches to the practice: first to establish stable clarity in the radiant appearance of the channels and chakras for a prolonged period of time; and not to do so. The former is the most effective approach. The [Indian] mahasiddha Lawapa[38] also gave the advice that we should cultivate the radiant appearance of the channels.

Here if one wishes to conjoin the practice with that of retaining the breath, one should do as explained earlier [with the breath technique instruction]. It, the physical exercises, and the meditation on the body as an empty shell, can be engaged in rotation. This should also be applied to what will come later.

Meditating by means of visualizing the mantric syllables

In the practice of the inner heat yoga one meditates on all four chakras. More precisely, one meditates upon the three energy channels, four chakras, and also a mantric syllable at each of the four chakras.

This is the instruction given in both *The Hevajra Root Tantra* (Skt. *Hevajra mula tantra*) and *The Sambhuta Explanatory Tantra* (Skt. *Samputa tantraraja tika*), as well as in other sources. Moreover, it is also the transmission handed down to us from many of the [Indian] mahasiddhas of old, including Krishnacharya himself.[39]

Generally speaking, the practice of envisioning the mantric syllables at the chakras can be done either elaborately or else simply.

In the former method, one visualizes a syllable at the center of each chakra, as well as on each of the petals. However, the oral instructions of this tradition do not elucidate this more elaborate process. Instead, they advocate that we should simply visualize a mantric syllable at the center of each of the four chakras. This is also the process taught in *The Sambhuta Explanatory Tantra* and in the writings of many of the Indian mahasiddhas.

Therefore solely to meditate on the *AH*-stroke mantric syllable at the navel chakra [as some teachers today recommend], or to meditate on the *AH*-stroke at the navel chakra together with *HAM* at the forehead chakra, is not sufficient. One should also bring in meditation on the syllables at the heart and throat chakras. This is important.

The manner of this meditation is as follows. One sits in the bodily posture described earlier. The place where the *AH*-stroke mantric syllable is to be visualized is the center of the central channel, just in front of the spinal column, at the place where the channel runs through the navel chakra. One should only meditate on the syllable as being at that point.

The process is as follows. One observes the navel chakra, known as "the wheel of emanation." At its center one envisions the *AH*-stroke syllable, standing upon a tiny moon cushion. It is in its Sanskrit form, which resembles the Tibetan character *shad* in the Tibetan classical script [i.e., the vertical stroke that divides Tibetan sentences]. It is red in color, and stands upright.

As for the syllable at the heart chakra, known as "the wheel of truth," which has eight petals, the place of this chakra is at the central channel just in front of the spine, at the point midway between the two nipples. One meditates only on the point at the center of the central channel. In this process of meditation one observes a tiny moon disk at the center of the chakra, and upon it a blue syllable *HUM*, its head pointing downward. One meditates that it has the power to cause the bodhimind substance to descend like falling snow.

Next one concentrates on the chakra known as "the wheel of enjoyment," which has sixteen petals. The place of this chakra is at the throat [i.e., behind the Adam's apple], and again the central channel runs through it, just in front of the spinal column. It is there that one places one's concentration, and observes a tiny moon disk, a tiny red syllable *OM* standing upright upon it.

Finally one focuses upon the chakra at the crown of the head, known as "the wheel of great ecstasy," which has thirty-two petals, the central channel running up the center of it. One observes a moon disk at its center, a white syllable *HAM* standing upon it, its head pointed downward.

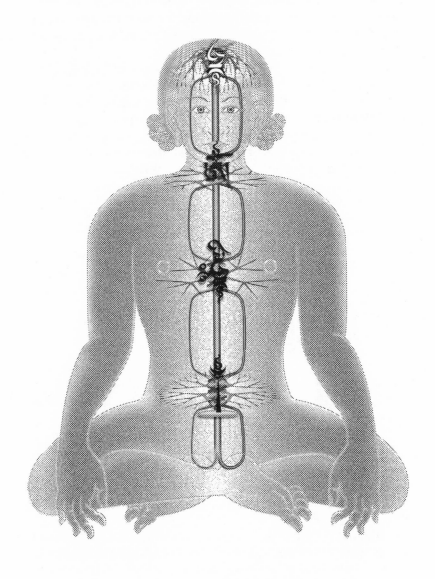

Channels, chakras and mantric syllables for the inner heat yoga

With all four of these chakras it is important to remember that the central channel runs through the center of them, and the side channels wrap around and constrict the central channel at the places of the chakras. It is important to conduct the meditations at the level of the knots, and to envision each mantric syllable as being at the center of the central channel. *The Sambhuta Explanatory Tantra* states,

> At the center of the heart is a lotus
> With eight petals, together with its essence;
> The channel that runs through its center
> Has the nature of a flame from a butterlamp
> And resembles the flower of the water tree
> Opened in bloom, petals stretched downward.
> Residing at its center is the hero,
> The size of a mustard seed,
> The indestructible syllable *HUM*,
> Causing the seed to fall like snow.

Here the expression "At the center, together with its essence" refers to the central channel. "Residing at its center... syllable *HUM*" indicates that one should practice the meditation at the center of the central channel. The same applies to the syllables in each of the other three chakras.

Although most oral transmissions [of this Six Yogas system] teach that one should meditate on the mantric syllables at the center of the chakras, in some it is not clearly taught that one should meditate only from within the center of the central channel. If this point is not emphasized and one meditates without doing so, the vital energies will not be drawn into the central channel. Consequently one will miss the essential purpose of the instruction.

As for the size of the mantric syllables, such as the syllable *HUM* [mentioned above in the quotation], it is a standard practice to visualize them as being the size of a mustard seed. However, the smaller that one can envision them, and the more clearly one can do so, the easier it becomes to draw the vital energies inside.

Although *The Sambhuta Explanatory Tantra* does not mention that the *AH*-stroke syllable [at the navel chakra] should be envisioned as having a tiny "ley-kor" [Tib. *klad kor*; i.e., sun-like circle] above it, *A Harvest of Oral Tradition Teachings* clearly states that it should. Likewise, the Chakrasamvara-related tantric text entitled *The Arising of Samvara Tantra* (Skt. *Samvarodaya tantra*) informs us that all four syllables should have all three elements of the crescent: the half moon, the drop, and the nada. They should be seen as melting the bodhimind substances like dewdrops flowing down. This is important for arousing the great ecstasy.

If the image can be held with radiance, this will help to prevent torpor from setting in during meditation, and will increase the clarity of one's samadhi.

The manner of holding the visualization in the mind is to do so as though one's entire conscious being had become immersed in the tiny image. The sense should not be as though we are in one place and are looking at the visualized image in another, but rather as though the mind apprehending the image had actually entered into and become utterly blended with it.

Whatever the state of realization induced by meditating in this way, to that same degree does the mind blend with the drop [of bodhimind substance]. This in turn renders the vital energies more easily gathered.

When one engages in the meditations it is important that in holding the image one does not apply either too much or too little mental effort. The former will result in mental agitation, and the latter in mental dullness. One should avoid these two pitfalls and hold to the image accordingly. Moreover, one should concentrate on the syllables of the upper three chakras for just a short period of time, and then dedicate most of the session to meditating on the *AH*-stroke syllable at the navel chakra.

Should the effort of envisioning the syllables as tiny in size remain difficult even after an extended application, then one can begin by visualizing them as large, and later simply reduce them in size in one's mind.

Meditating like this on the inner heat yoga has the purpose of inducing the four blisses. To effect this, first the bodhimind substance in the channels must be melted, and together with the vital energies must be brought to the chakra at the crown. This generates the first bliss, known simply as "bliss." The substances in the channels again flow, and then collect at the chakra at the throat; the second bliss, known as "supreme bliss," is aroused. Again the substances flow, and then collect at the chakra at the heart; the third bliss, known as "special bliss," arises. Fourthly, the energies collect at the chakra at the navel; the bliss known as "innate bliss" is induced.

It is important in each of these four chakra meditations that the mind is held on the mantric syllable at the center of each individual chakra, which is [located at] the center of the central channel, called *avadhuti*, as this makes it easier to collect the vital energies [at the specific chakra being meditated upon].

At each of the four sites a unique experience of bliss is aroused, and one must cultivate the ability to consciously recognize these in one's own experience.

The bodhimind substance that resides in the upper chakra is melted and brought to each of the four chakras, where it must be retained. If one cannot hold it in the chakras for a prolonged period of time one will not be able to appreciate the uniqueness of each of the four experiences of bliss. In particular, one will not be able to discern the uniqueness of the fourth, the innate bliss.

If one can achieve stability in the technique of holding the mind at the four chakras for prolonged periods, one will be able to control the movement of the bodhimind substance for an according degree of time. This is an important key to progress.

Moreover, if one can fix the mind firmly on the syllable *HAM* at the crown chakra, this will cause the force of the white male substance to increase, for this is the seat of the white bodhimind substance. Similarly, if one can fix the mind firmly on the syllable at the throat chakra, which is the site where the force of blood [i.e., red female substance] is retained and released in the rasana channel, this will increase the power of the inner heat, which arises at the navel chakra, and in turn is the force used to direct the drop. In addition, this experience will enhance one's ability to practice dream yoga [dreams being linked to the throat chakra]. Thirdly, holding the mind with stability on the syllable *HUM* at the heart chakra, which is the supreme site from which the clear light consciousness is generated, intensifies the strength of the clear light consciousness during both sleeping and waking states. Fourthly, when one retains the mind at the *AH*-stroke syllable at the navel chakra, which is the site at which the channel lalana will increase the retaining and releasing power of the male genetic substance, the white bodhimind substance will flow from the navel chakra and will be diffused into the entire body, which is an important key to progress. Moreover, the navel chakra is the special site at which abides the fire of the inner heat, which is the force used to melt the bodhimind substance.

It is important that we understand the process of correctly meditating upon these chakras and the mantric syllables associated with them.

As the Indian mahasiddha Lawapa advised, we should persist in the meditation until the mantric syllables appear with utter clarity and radiance.

Meditating by means of engaging the vase breathing technique

One begins by generally visualizing the energy channels, as was explained previously, and holding the mind on that image, making the awareness firm at the place in the central channel where the three channels meet. One then observes the four mantric syllables at the center of the central channel [at the sites of the four chakras], again placing awareness firmly on the *AH*-stroke mantric syllable four fingerwidths below the navel at the center of the central channel. As this is the place at which the vital energies are drawn into the central channel by means of mental application, placing the mind here will definitely encourage the process of collecting the vital energies.

The Arising of Samvara Tantra as well as *The Sambhuta Explanatory Tantra* associated with both the Chakrasamvara and Hevajra tantric cycles recommend that in the yoga of arousing the inner heat one should meditate on the mantric syllable in the fourth chakra. They do not mention doing so in conjunction with uniting the vital energies by means of the vase breathing technique. The tantric writings of the Indian mahasiddhas Krishnacharya, Lawapa and Padma are similar in this respect.

Likewise, most of the important oral tradition lineages on the practice of the completion stage tantric yogas do not mention meditation with the vase breathing technique at this point. They simply state that when one meditates on the basis of fully understanding the process of mental focusing as explained earlier, that by itself will draw the life-sustaining energies into the central channel and cause the inner fires to blaze with strength. This in turn will melt the bodhimind substance, and the experiences of the four blisses will definitely occur.

However, many Tibetan lamas holding the oral tradition have advised that one would do well to supplement the process of visualizing the channels, chakras and mantric syllables with the vase breathing technique. This quickens the arousal of the inner heat. Therefore it is explained here.

The technique itself has four phases: drawing in the airs; filling like a vase; compressing the airs; and releasing them like an arrow. These are the four special features of the vase breathing method as taught by the lamas of the past.

Some holders of oral traditions have commented in their writings that the source of this method is *The Four Seats Tantra*. There is a danger in making such claims without first closely scrutinizing that tantra.

The vase breathing technique begins with sitting in meditation in the posture explained earlier. As for the time for practice, the manual of glorious Pakmo Drupa comments that although some lamas recommend the occasion when the breath is flowing evenly through both nostrils, in fact any time of the day or night is an appropriate time for the practice. However, when one commences the training, because breath is associated with vajra speech, i.e., the communicative principle of enlightenment, an auspicious time to begin is when the vital energy known as "lotus protector" is most easily caused to rise. This is stated in the commentary to *The Arising of Samvara Tantra* entitled *The Lotus Receptacle* (Skt. *Padmini*).[40]

As for how one takes in the breath, one does not do so through the mouth, but rather through the nostrils; and one does not apply force, but rather gently draws in a long, deep breath.

In the process called "filling the vase" one holds the air inside, not allowing any to leave, and presses it down. One imagines that the breath enters the two side channels—*rasana* and *lalana*—and fills them out, like an empty intestine inflated with air. Both side channels are envisioned as becoming filled in this way.

The process of compressing the air is as follows. After the side channels have become filled one meditates that the air from both of them flows into the central channel. One swallows without making any sound and retains the air in this way, while pressing down with the abdomen. Simultaneously from below one draws in air gently from the two lower apertures [i.e., anus and sexual passage] to the site of the *AH*-stroke mantric syllable. Meditating in this way, hold the air inside for as long as possible.

Here the verse commentary of glorious Pakmo Drupa recommends that one meditate on the air as flowing from the two side channels, *rasana* and *lalana*, into the central channel. This is the application of "filling." Retain the air if possible. If not possible, then after the period of a cycle of finger snaps one releases the air slowly, using whatever is left inside for the dissolving process. However, Pakmo Drupa's prose commentary explains the process in accordance with what was said earlier.[41]

Although glorious Pakmo Drupa thus presents two quite different instructions, the only real difference occurs in one of the four phases.

His instructions on drawing in the airs, retaining them and then ex-pelling them are the same in each case. As for the process of "filling," the air that has been inhaled fills the *rasana* and *lalana* channels; for the compressing, the air in these two channels is envisioned as flow-ing into the central channel. The air in the side channels is compressed, forcing it to flow into and fill the central channel.[42]

With this meditation on the vase breathing technique at the navel chakra, some teachers state that one should not draw up the airs from below, but should solely press down from above [with the abdomen]. Others say that one first presses down from above for some time, and then afterwards draws up from below three times.

These theories fail to appreciate the dynamic involved in vase breathing at the navel chakra. One of the key elements in the medita-tion is that one wants to redirect the life-sustaining energies flowing above the navel, and also the eliminating energies from below the navel, and blend these two.

The Arising of Samvara Tantra explains it as follows,

> The energies that course above and below
> Through the mind are brought to a kiss.

Thus this tantra states that the vital energies from above and below are to be brought together in a kiss through the application. There-fore one should both press down the airs from above and draw them up from below. One should not do so simultaneously, but rather first do the one and then the other. Unless there is a special reason for doing otherwise [such as a health problem], then one first presses down the air from above into the navel chakra, and then draws up the lower airs from below to that same site, thus pressing the two together. One simply does both of these applications one time each; there is no need for doing so three times each [as some recommend].

The fourth phase, that of releasing like an arrow, instructs that in releasing the breath one should do so gently and quietly, imagining that it comes up the central channel. However, one does not visualize it as leaving by the crown aperture [as some teachers advise].

Thus the airs from above and below are drawn to the navel chakra. At this point, however, it is not appropriate to visualize that the en-tire body is filled with pure vital energies [as some teachers have sug-gested], nor that solely the heart and throat chakras of the upper re-gions are filled [as others have suggested].

Instead one concentrates upon the *AH*-stroke mantric syllable [at the navel chakra], and at that place of meditation brings the upper and lower airs into a kiss. This is a supreme key.

In fact we need to possess two keys: that for bringing together the life-sustaining energies, which have been drawn into the central channel, and the eliminating [or, alternatively, the downward-moving] energies, into a kiss at that place [i.e., at the site of the mantric syllable at the center of the central channel, at the location of the navel chakra]; and, secondly, we need the radiant clarity of the appearance of the tiny mantric syllable, as was meditated upon previously.

Here it is said that when the side channels *rasana* and *lalana* have their lower apertures open, that of the central channel will remain closed. Conversely, when that of the central channel is opened, those of the side channels will remain closed.

One visualizes that through the vase breathing meditation the flow of the vital energies of the side channels is prevented from escaping, and instead is redirected into the central channel. The meditation has these two aspects. When the technique has reached maturity one gains the power to actually draw the energies into the central channel.

As for how to retain the airs, and the duration of the sessions, here the instruction of glorious Pakmo Drupa states,

> At first concentrate on cleaning the energy channel system, and try not to force the energies. Press the airs [while holding the breath] just so long as a sense of forcing is absent, applying just the appropriate intensity.

As said here, until some progress has been made one should apply gentleness in the method [of breath retention and the according meditation on bringing the upper and lower energies together at the navel chakra]. Do not force the upper part of the body, and do not draw up from below too forcefully.

The duration of the sessions should not be such that sensations of discomfort come to dominate the experience. To force things will not induce the energies to enter into the central channel. Even should it cause the energies to enter the navel chakra for a moment, they will not remain there, and will leave. Moreover, although retaining the energies outside the chakra may produce some heat and ecstasy, such as the ability to raise the body temperature, or sensations of bliss, this will not help to bring the vital energies into the central channel.

For example, when one first takes up the practice of meditation one can only hold the mind on its object for a moment, and then it slips away. It does not abide by its own inclination. Only when one has arrived at a particular level in the training will it remain of its own impetus. Similarly, although the energies may occasionally enter the navel chakra through forceful practice, their inclination is to flow and not to remain, and thus one will not be able to retain them. They will not naturally remain; and if one attempts to force them, they cannot be retained at the desired place. Dangerous obstacles can be incurred, and not the slightest desirable effect achieved.

When the energies begin naturally to remain, then one can extend the duration of the application. Carefully and skillfully observing the process will bring the ability to know if the energies will naturally remain or not, and if they can be retained at the desired place.

The time for practicing the vase breathing technique is on an empty stomach, or when the food is well digested. Meditate in sessions that are not too long in duration, taking occasional rests. Do not do so for long sessions without taking a break.

When skill in the vase breathing technique is stabilized, one engages in the technique in conjunction with visualizing the four mantric syllables at the center of the chakras at the navel, heart, throat and crown. The syllables are at the center of the central channel, the side channels coiled around it [at these locations], the apertures as described earlier. One clearly visualizes the mantric syllables *AM, HUM, OM* and *HAM* in this way.

Then the energies residing in the chakra at the secret place cause the *AH*-stroke syllable at the navel chakra, which is in nature the inner fire, to blaze with light. This light rises up the central channel *avadhuti* and melts the other three syllables, *HAM, OM* and *HUM* [respectively at the crown, throat and heart chakras]. These melt and fall into the syllable *AM* [at the navel chakra].[43] The four become of one inseparable nature. One then fixes the mind on the drop [formed by this fusion], the nature of which is the innate ecstasy. If one can do so, then from the drop comes the tongue of a tiny flame of the inner heat. One fixes the mind on it.

Light from this flame rises up the central channel, where it melts the drop of white bodhimind substance abiding within the crown chakra. This drips down like nectar, filling the *AM*-stroke mantric syllable at the navel chakra. One meditates single-pointedly on the

AM-stroke, until the signs of stability arise. When meditative stability has been achieved then the radiance of the light from the inner fire will illuminate the inside and outside of one's body, as well as one's dwelling place and so forth, rendering them as transparent as a piece of *kyurura* fruit held in the hand.

It is important to meditate like that, keeping the mind on the tiny flame. Doing so is said to render one's samadhi more subtle, and to encourage quick and easy fulfillment of one's meditative power.

Having meditated in this way, how to cause the vital energies to enter, abide, and dissolve within the central channel

By means of the three previous meditations, one arrives at the threshold wherein one can successfully apply the technology for causing the vital energies to enter into the central channel.

What are the unmistaken signs that occur? This is an important question. Numerous signs are mentioned in various traditions, but many of these seem to be superficial. The convincing signs are as follows.

After completing a session, one checks to discern the nostril through which the airs are mainly passing. One then engages in the bodily posture and mental application.

After some time of applying the practice, one observes the nostrils, and draws in several breaths in order to see how evenly the breath is flowing through the two nostrils. Should it naturally flow evenly in both without any force being exerted from one's side, this is a sign that the strength of the yoga has transported one to the stage wherein the energies can be drawn into the central channel. However, if this sign only happens once or twice, it is not very certain.

The best sign is that, if there is no other obstruction, the airs flow through both nostrils, and the two flows are of equal strength, without one being strong and the other weak. This can be regarded as a sign that one has reached the stage at which the energies have begun to enter the central channel. However, it is not the case that, once it has entered, the flow of breath will not alternate between the nostrils. That is the entering. As for the process of causing it to remain, one meditates with great strength, and the breath becomes weak. At the end one observes carefully; the breath becomes increasingly subtle, and eventually stops altogether. Concerning this experience Jetsun Milarepa stated,

> When the energies in *rasana* and *lalana*
> Enter into the central channel *avadhuti*,
> Ecstasy [is experienced].

And also,

> When the breath no longer comes and goes, ecstasy;
> When one completely cuts off the flow, ecstasy.

After stopping the flow there are two possible situations: in the first of these the process of dissolving the energies is easy, and in the second it is more difficult. If it is difficult, then for a moment one feels as though one's stomach is filled with air, but the sensation soon ceases. Then there is a sensation of heat from the residences of the inner fire in the navel and secret chakras. This induces melting [of the substances], and an according experience of ecstasy.

However, this stopping of the subtle breath may occur without one having actually dispelled subtle meditative torpor. Someone with this obstacle can accomplish stoppage of the breath.

Without having the skill of focusing at the center of the navel chakra, merely doing the vase breathing technique will not cause the energies to remain, and they will dissipate to other sites. Such a situation can happen; there is no flow of breath, but also no retention of the energies in the chakra. There is neither entering nor dissolving. One must understand these distinctions in the training.

As for the duration of time that the air/energies should be retained by the vase practice, here *The Arising of Samvara Tantra* states,

> By practicing the vase breathing as instructed,
> One sits with legs crossed in the vajra posture,
> With the hand rubs thrice,
> And then snaps the fingers six times.
> Until the breath can be retained
> For thirty-six cycles of this measurement,
> Persist in practice of the vase breathing technique.
> Those who can do three times thirty-six
> Are able to retain the airs for more than 108 cycles.

In accordance with what is recommended above, one places one's right palm on the left, strokes three times, and then snaps the fingers six times. The best practitioner can repeat 108 cycles of this measurement; the intermediate can repeat seventy-two; and the smallest can repeat it thirty-six times while holding the breath. All three of these [have reached the stage at which they] are able to triumph over death.[44]

Having brought in the energies, the methods of arousing the four blisses

This is explained under three headings: the nature of the signs that arise, together with the blazing of the inner fire; the manner of generating the four blisses by means of melting the bodhimind substances; and the manner of meditating upon the innate wisdom.

The nature of the signs that arise, and the blazing of the inner fire

One places the mind at the center of the navel chakra and brings the life-sustaining energies into the central channel. This gives rise to the signs.

The manner in which the signs arise is described by the [Indian] mahasiddha Lawapa,

> The first sign is like a mirage,
> The second like a wisp of smoke,
> The third like the flickering of fireflies,
> The fourth like a glowing butterlamp,
> And the fifth a formless sign
> Resembling a sky free of clouds.

The first of the signs is like a mirage, or like a hallucination or illusory appearance. The next four signs are increasingly clear. They resemble respectively a mirage, smoke, and so forth.

These days there are three popular interpretations of these signs. Some people say that they do not literally appear as described. Others say that the experience is merely a reflection of the stability or wavering of the mind that perceives them; and still others state that the signs, such as smoke and so forth, do actually appear as described. This last is best.

Actually, there will be a variation in the force with which the energies collect at different times, as well as in the depth of the experience, the stability or lack of it, and so forth. Hence there is no single way of describing the visions. For example, one must make a difference between the experience of the signs such as smoke and so forth as apprehended by someone who has applied the special techniques for bringing the energies into the central channel and then held the awareness there, and as apprehended by someone who has not done this, but rather has generated the signs merely by strenuous application of holding awareness of non-thought.

In the former of these two cases, an important phase of the practice is that of arresting the energy of the earth element. It is said that three signs manifest when it has become somewhat redirected. Likewise, the energies that flow outside through the doors of the sensory powers must be arrested and redirected; different signs appear when this process is initiated, when it has become somewhat established, and when these energies have been somewhat redirected into the central channel. Then there is the stoppage of the energy flow associated with the attainment of a higher plane, and the stages of special signs that occur with the mere stoppage of energies.

When the signs arise due to the dissolutions and the process of bringing the energies into the central channel, then all five, from the mirage to the sky without clouds, will occur without interruption. The earth energies dissolve into those of water, and the mirage-like sign is beheld; the water energies dissolve into those of fire, and there is the sign of smoke; the fire energies dissolve into those of wind, and the sign of sparks, like flickering fireflies, appears. Then the energy that carries conceptual thought dissolves into mind, and there is an appearance like that of the light of a butterlamp undisturbed by wind.

It is said that the strength of the experiences indicated by these signs will eventually carry one to the stage wherein the realization of mahamudra is achieved.

The inner heat that can be aroused is of various types. For example, there is the inner heat in the central channel, that is first aroused in the chakras at the navel and secret place, and there is the inner heat that blazes and increases outside the central channel. Secondly, there is the heat that is aroused from the depth of the body, and also the heat aroused at the surface, between the skin and flesh. Then there is the heat [that seems to pervade] narrow [areas of the body], and the heat that seems to pervade large areas, as aroused on initial stages of practice. Then there is the heat that rises slowly, and the heat that arises quickly. Also, there is the heat that seems thick, and the heat that seems thin. In each of these pairs, the first is better than the second. The second indicates an inferior experience.

Due to these differences there are also different levels of arousing the blisses. In turn, there is either the special inner heat, and there is mere warmth. Then there is the bliss induced merely by controlling the energies, and also the bliss induced by melting the substances. One should understand these distinctions.

When the special inner heat is ignited, the bodhimind substances will accordingly be melted. Here no ill side-effects will occur as a result of upsetting the balance of the elements. Conversely, in the production of a less exalted heat one will not necessarily produce the melting of the drops. Bile and sexual craving may be increased in the body [causing an imbalance], and instead of blissfulness one may experience sensations of unpleasant heat.

If the igniting of the heat is done properly, then the white bodhimind substance will be melted and increased. The melting and dropping of this white drop will cause the inner heat of the red bodhimind substance to grow in strength.

How the bodhimind substances are melted and the four blisses induced

The bodhimind substance is melted and descends [from its site in the crown chakra]. When it arrives in each of the four chakras it gives rise respectively to the four descending blisses.

The Diamond Rosary Tantra (Skt. *Vajramala tantra*) explains the process as follows,

> Then there is the explanation of the arising of the experiences:
> From the wheel of great ecstasy, the chakra at the crown,
> The eperience known as "bliss" arises;
> From the wheel of enjoyment, the chakra at the throat,
> The "supreme bliss" is aroused;
> From the wheel of truth, the chakra at the heart,
> The "inexpressible bliss" occurs;
> And from the wheel of emanation, the chakra at the navel,
> The "innate bliss" is induced.
> Thus are the four blisses experienced.

As said here, the bodhimind substance leaves the crown chakra and arrives at the throat chakra; "bliss" is experienced. It leaves the throat chakra and arrives at the heart; "the supreme bliss" is experienced. It leaves the heart chakra and arrives at the navel; "the special bliss" is aroused. Finally it leaves the navel chakra and comes to the chakra at the secret place, the tip of the jewel; the "innate bliss" is experienced.

As for how the four blisses are experienced when the drop is brought back up the central channel and through the chakras, this is explained in the same text as follows:

> At the wheel of emanation, bliss;
> At the wheel of truth, supreme bliss;
> At the wheel of enjoyment, inexpressible bliss;
> And at the wheel of great ecstasy, the innate bliss:
> Thus are the four upward-moving blisses experienced in
>   reverse order.

Here we can see that the process follows the pattern of the descending blisses, except in reverse. The same explanation is given in *The Mark of Mahamudra* (Skt. *Mahamudra tilika*).

The four descending and rising blisses can each be distinguished into four each. These are known as "the sixteen phases of the moon." When the distinction is made on the basis of the sun, then each of the four can be subdivided into three, making "the twelve phases of the sun." The same text says,

> Like phases of the moon
> Are the sixteen drops of ecstasy.
> They should be understood as being
> In the nature of the sixteen vowel sounds [of the Sanskrit
>   alphabet].
> From the stages of experience in the four chakras
> Are said to arise the twelve phases of the sun;
> Thus do the teachings describe it.

Here when the white bodhimind substance moves down and then up through the central channel and four chakras it draws red bodhimind substance with it. Thus in each of the chakras there are four elements of experience, and each of these gives rise to a unique experience of ecstasy. These are "the sixteen phases of the moon." Similarly, the bliss experienced in each of the four chakras can be distinguished into three degrees of intensity, known as small, medium and great. These are "the twelve phases of the sun."

One must learn to distinguish these sixteen and twelve in the continuum of one's own experience.

In general it is said that the descending blisses are less strong than those aroused by bringing the drop back up the channel through the chakras.

When drawing up the bodhimind substance from below, the bliss experienced will not become stable until the control of the chakra at the crown has been firmly established. When control over the crown chakra becomes firm, then the experience of the blisses becomes firm. The same text says,

> When the mind based on the vital energies flows,
> The bodhimind substance moves back up the channel
> And the drop comes to the center of the lotus.
> If it can be stabilized there,
> Then the lord of ecstasy will not leave,
> Just like a pot without a hole

Will not allow water in it to escape.
At that time the experience of ecstasy becomes stable,
And that firmness in turn arouses the innate ecstasy.
Consequently the state of inexhaustible buddhahood
Shall certainly be accomplished by that yogi.

As *A Harvest of Oral Tradition Teachings* points out, here "mind" refers to the white drop; "flows" refers to the reversing process; and "becomes stable" refers to the crown chakra.

Various oral traditions state that practice of the inner heat meditation causes sensations of warmth to arise, and based on this warmth the bodhimind substances are melted inside the channels. From the melting comes ecstasy, and from the ecstasy arises a state of beyond-conceptuality consciousness. However, merely this depth of understanding does not account for the importance in general of the four descending and four rising-from-below blisses, nor in particular the importance of dwelling within the innate bliss.

The explanation above, which deals with the two sets of four blisses, is in accord with what is taught in the original tantric scriptures, as well as in the treatises written by the [Indian] mahasiddhas.

In general, ecstasy may be experienced either by meditators who melt the bodhimind substance by means of the yogas described earlier, or by those who have not meditated in this way. In both cases there will be the kindling of the inner fires at the navel and secret place chakras, and from this heat the bodhimind substances will be caused to move; but this does not necessarily mean that the flow will be contained within the central channel.

Thus some practitioners experience melting of the substances and also the blisses, even though they have not generated the ability to direct the energies into the central channel. This frequently occurs when using certain techniques of meditation that focus on particular points of the body.

Once the bodhimind substance begins to move one should establish firm control over it before it arrives at the vajra jewel chakra, or it will prove very difficult to retain. From the beginning one applies the outer and inner methods to cause the bodhimind substance to move downward. While it is passing through the upper chakras, and before it arrives at the jewel chakra, one must exert strong methods to control it. Similarly, the moment it arrives at the jewel chakra one must exert this control forcefully in order to halt its movement.

Here one must take care, for if these methods are applied too vigorously the drop may be incorrectly diffused into the bodily paths, causing any of a variety of illnesses. A number of methods of correctly diffusing the drop have been discussed by various lamas. What we want here is to discern the process of dissolving the vital energies into *avadhuti*, the central channel, and thus melting the bodhimind substance, while preventing it from melting in other ways. A discussion of crucial distinctions, such as the ease or difficulty of retaining control of the drop, often is not found [in Tibetan manuals].

One must understand the principles of how much force to apply in the controlling process, precisely when such application is required and not required, and how to avoid incurring physical illnesses through incorrectly diffusing the drop into the bodily paths. These are not discussed with sufficient clarity [in some traditions of tantric practice].

The main purpose behind these meditations that ignite the inner heat and melt the bodhimind substances is to arouse the innate bliss. In this process one melts the bodhimind substances and causes them to descend. In general, when they arrive at the chakras below the navel, and in particular when they arrive at the jewel chakra, they must be prevented from being ejaculated, and must be held at that site for some time. Otherwise one will not experience the authentic innate bliss. To arouse the innate bliss of the completion stage yogas one must first dissolve and then retain the vital energies in the central channel.

If the experience is based on dissolving the vital energies into the central channel and the melting of the bodhimind substance, then when the drop arrives at the tip of the jewel one is able to restrain it from being ejaculated for as long as it takes to induce the complete experience of the innate ecstasy. As the bodhimind substance gradually descends from the crown chakra it sublimates the force of the energies. As a result, by the time it arrives at the jewel chakra it has already arrested the flow of the subtle bodily energy that causes ejaculation.

For some people it is difficult to withdraw the energies but easy to produce the melting. For others it is difficult to melt the substances but easy to withdraw the energies.

The inner heat practice can sometimes effect a quick melting, but unless the melting is subtle in intensity it will be difficult for one to control the drop. If control is not established when the drop moves through the upper chakras, it will prove exceedingly difficult to initiate this control when it arrives at the lower chakras. And even if some control is established [at that late phase] it will be difficult to correctly diffuse it, increasing the danger of physical illnesses being created from side-effects. When the dissolving of the energies occurs correctly as in the process described earlier, none of these problems arise.

Sometimes in bringing the vital energies under control an accidental melting of the substances occurs before the dissolution of the energies has been effected, and the blisses spontaneously arise. How should one do the stopping and diffusing?

Simply try to slow down the process of melting, and without applying too much force in the meditation bring the drop back up to the crown chakra. Then diffuse the melting throughout the various channels and sites. Practicing in this way, one eventually will be able to control the drop even during a strong experience of melting.

Also, if a strong experience of melting suddenly occurs and one is unable to do as described above, then revert to the visualization of oneself as the mandala deity. Sit in the vajra posture, cross the hands in front of the chest, wrathfully elevate the gaze of the two eyes, contract the toes and fingers, place the mind on the mantric syllable *HAM* in the crown chakra, which now is seen as standing upright [unlike in the usual visualization process], and wrathfully yet slowly recite the mantric syllable *HUM* twenty-one times. Meditate that the drop thus travels back up the central channel in front of the spine, and returns to the crown chakra from whence it had descended. Then engage in a soft exercise of the vase breathing technique and also shake the body gently. Meditate that the bodhimind substances are diffused throughout the appropriate sites of the channels. Repeat this process several times.

The manner of meditating upon the innate wisdom

As explained earlier in the description of the descending process, the bodhimind substance is melted and arrives at the chakra at the tip of the jewel. If one can retain it without ejaculation, the innate ecstasy will be aroused. At that time one must engage mindfulness of the view of emptiness to be ascertained, and must place the mind firmly there. Rest within the inseparable ecstasy and [wisdom of] emptiness. Even if you do not have a profound understanding of the emptiness doctrine, at least avoid all distractions and rest in the singular ecstasy of the experience until the absorption becomes stable, mixing this with the beyond-conceptuality consciousness.

While doing this, retain the bodhimind substance in the jewel chakra for some time. Then reverse it, bringing it back up to the crown chakra. This gives rise to the "rising-from-below" innate wisdom. Identify this clearly in the awareness, and then fix the mind in the sphere of ecstasy conjoined with [the wisdom of] emptiness. If this is impossible, then simply try to rest the mind in the ecstasy and to blend this with the beyond-conceptuality consciousness. Remain in that state for as long as possible. This is the manner in which one cultivates the experience during formal meditation sessions.

As for how to cultivate the training during the post-meditation periods, one should note that in general merely the presence of the innate ecstasy in meditation does not mean that the realization will automatically carry over into the post-meditation periods. The ecstasy that was experienced will not necessarily become manifest in [perception of] the objects that appear during everyday activities. That by itself is not enough. During the post-meditation periods one must consciously cultivate mindfulness of the experience of ecstasy and emptiness, and stamp all objects and events that appear and occur with the seal of this ecstasy and emptiness. This application causes a special ecstasy to be ignited, which one should foster.

Although this approach is not clearly elucidated in some of the oral traditions, it is explained in detail in the Marpa lineage as transmitted to Lama Ngokpa. Also, it is taught in several of the original tantras, including *The Hevajra Root Tantra*. Therefore it is important not to ignore it.

Thus one practices both during meditation sessions and in the post-meditation periods. In this way one proceeds by conjoining meditation on the inner fire, uniting the vital energies, and invoking the four blisses.

The external condition of relying upon a karmamudra

Here both oneself and the mudra should be beings of highest capacity, and should have received the pure empowerments. Both should be learned in the root and branch guidelines of tantric practice, and have the ability to maintain them well. Both should be skilled in the sadhana of the mandala cycle, and mature in practicing four daily sessions of yoga.

Also, they should be skilled in the sixty-four ways of sexual play as described in *The Treatise on Bliss* (Skt. *Kama shastra*). They should be mature in meditation upon the doctrine of emptiness; be experienced in the techniques for inducing the four blisses in general and the innate wisdom awareness in particular; and be able to control the melted drops and prevent them from escaping outside.

Such are the characteristics required of the practitioners as described in the original tantras and also in the treatises of the [Indian] mahasiddhas.[45]

There are those, of course, who claim that all these characteristics need not be present, and that still the practice will be profound. They quote various oral tradition lineages as their source. I can only say that to practice on that basis is exceedingly unwise, and easily opens the door to the lower realms.

On this point the text *The Arising of Heruka Tantra* (Skt. *Shri heruka abhyudaya tantra*) clearly states,

> To call non-yoga a yogic Dharma,
> To rely on a mudra in order to cross in that way,
> And to pretend that non-wisdom is wisdom
> Without a doubt only leads to the hell realms.

Therefore as said here, those wishing to engage physically in the sexual yogas should be qualified. To practice on any other basis presents great dangers. One should understand this well.

Those not qualified to take up the karmamudra practices should instead engage in prolonged meditation upon a jnanamudra [i.e., a visualized consort], such as the mandala dakinis Nairatmya and Vajrayogini. When the practice achieves stability and the visualization arises with total presence and radiance, one can enter into sexual union with this visualized consort and arouse the four blisses. The innate ecstasy emerges, and one unites this with [the wisdom of] emptiness, thus blending mindfulness of the view [of emptiness] with the great ecstasy. This is the experience known as ecstasy and emptiness in union.

If one is unable to do this, one simply relies on ecstasy and cultivates the samadhi that rests one-pointedly within that bliss.

Having aroused the four blisses, how to engage in the meditations on the
illusory body and clear light doctrines

This is explained under two headings: the general principles of
how, in reliance upon the inner heat yoga, one meditates on the remaining stages of the path; and the meditations of those particular
paths.

The general principles of how, in reliance upon the inner heat doctrine, one
meditates upon the remaining stages of the path

In this tradition [i.e., the Six Yogas of Naropa] the teachings on
how the inner heat yoga is used to bring the vital energies into the
central channel are very clear.

However, the tradition is somewhat unclear on how, once the energies have been drawn into the *avadhuti* channel, one engages in the
meditations on the illusory body and clear light doctrines. Although
it seems quite difficult to subtly analyze these two yogas I would like
to say something in order to give an appreciation of this extraordinary oral transmission.

As was pointed out earlier, the doctrines of the illusory body and
clear light yogas are said to be based upon the Guhyasamaja Tantra,
and also the oral tradition of the Guhyasamaja tantric system known
as the Arya Cycle. According to this latter, which is the transmission
of Nagarjuna and his disciples, for as long as the vital energies have
not been drawn into the central channel and caused to abide and dissolve, one will not be able to generate the samadhi of the threefold
experience of "appearance," "proximity" and "proximate attainment"
that precedes the accomplishment of mind refinement; and it is from
the state of vital energies and consciousness that have generated the
complete signs of the wisdom awareness of final mind refinement
that the qualified illusory body can be engaged.[46]

This is clear from what is said in the oral tradition of the Guhyasamaja Tantra coming from Lama Marpa. It is also clear in Lama
Marpa's transmission of the five completion stage yogas of the
Guhyasamaja system, as embodied in the text *Elucidation of the Sum-*
mary of the Five Stages (Skt. *Pancha kramartha baskarana nama*); and it is
clear in the oral tradition of that Five Stages transmission.

Thus although the basic principles of the illusory body and clear
light yogas are not clearly stated here [in the Six Yogas of Naropa
transmission], it seems that we should understand them in the context of the Guhyasamaja Arya Cycle doctrines.

Here the tradition of Lama Marpa is based on the text *Elucidation of the Summary of the Five Stages,* wherein we read,

> First one experiences the hallucination-like sign
> That arises with the halo of five lights.
> Secondly is a moon-like sign,
> And thirdly a sign like that of sunlight.
> Then is a sign like pre-dawn, and the attainment.

And also,

> Arising solely from energy and mind,
> The illusory body becomes manifest.

The first vision is like moonlight shining in a cloudless sky. This is the stage called "appearance" [mentioned above]. Next there is a vision like that of sunlight glimmering in the sky; this is the stage of "proximity." Then there is a vision of darkness, like the sky in early morning, with neither sun nor moon; this is the stage known as "proximate attainment." After these three have occurred, the subtle energies and consciousness of the state of mind refinement give rise to the illusory body, radiant with light.

These are the principles on which the illusory body doctrine [of Lama Marpa's tradition of Guhyasamaja] is based; but we do not see them discussed in this tradition [i.e., the Six Yogas].

Instead there is a discussion of an unpurified illusory body that is linked to the practice of observing one's image reflected in a mirror as a means of cutting off the coarse conceptual mind, such as thoughts of pleasure or displeasure at likes and dislikes. Then there is a discussion of a purified illusory body, which is linked to the practice of meditating upon the illusory nature of one's own body envisioned as that of a mandala deity, which induces a state of one-tasteness that does not discriminate between likes and dislikes.

Yet these two ["purified" and "unpurified" as described above] are only "illusory bodies" in a general sense common to both highest tantra and other paths. They are to be distinguished from the "unpurified illusory body" that is the third stage [of the Guhyasamaja five-stage system], known as "the hidden essence of illusory nature"; and the "purified illusory body" that is the fifth stage, also known as "the illusory body of the stage of great unification." It seems that this distinction is not even roughly made here.[47]

The actual illusory body doctrine is exclusive to highest yoga tantra. The first "illusory body" described above [i.e., observing one's image

in a mirror, etc.] does not even really qualify as a general-nature illusory essence [i.e., it is common to sutra teachings]; and the second
one [i.e., meditating on the illusory nature of oneself as a mandala
deity] is also found in the three lower classes of tantras [and hence is
not even exclusive to highest yoga tantra].

Mention is made of the practice having the effect of overcoming
the concepts of attraction and aversion, and thus equalizing them.
This actually refers to bringing together innate great ecstasy with the
wisdom of emptiness that cuts to the heart of the Middle View. This
is the principal meditation to be cultivated during formal sessions.
One should understand these two factors well [i.e., ecstasy and wis-
dom] and cultivate them.

When one arises from meditation sessions, the force of the meditative experience will carry over [into the post-meditation period], causing all that appears to arise with the presence of an illusion.

Actually, from the time of the first stage [i.e., the generation stage,
the beginning level of tantric training], a principal practice in the post-
meditation periods is to take all events and transport them into the
mandala deity activities. By means of this, an awareness of the illusory mandala deity and its non-inherent nature arises. Here that
awareness manifests automatically.

Some oral instruction lineages of the Guhyasamaja oral tradition
coming from Lama Marpa suggest that we place an image of the
mandala deity in front of a mirror and gaze at it, while meditating
that it is one's own image appearing as a reflection of the deity. They
comment that this is an oral tradition teaching for enhancing the radiant appearance of oneself as the mandala deity at the time of practicing the generation stage yogas. They also quote the oral tradition
from [Marpa's disciple] Lama Tsur, which comments that during the
secret empowerment an image of Vajrasattva is reflected in a mirror
and the disciples are instructed to observe it and reflect upon the non-
inherent nature of the illusory form of the mandala deity. These practices, they state, are to be brought into play here. They extract these
interpretations from *The Five Stages* without knowing the exact meaning of the words of that text.

I have explained these points extensively in my writings on the
instructions of the Arya Cycle of Guhyasamaja doctrines. None of
these doctrines were missing from the original oral tradition teachings of the Marpa transmission on the illusory body [even though

they are missing from most transmissions today]. I discuss this issue in the text mentioned above.

Moreover, although in this oral tradition we do find the doctrines of the "great union" on both levels of "in training" and "beyond training," and also the doctrines of the four states of appearance, proximity, proximate attainment and clear light, [it is helpful to refer to the Arya Cycle of the Guhyasamaja Tantra for greater detail on a number of points, in particular:] the methods of first producing the illusory body from subtle energy and subtle consciousness; and, having produced that illusory body, how one generates the four emptinesses, such as of appearance, proximity, etc., for the process of immersing the illusory body in the actual clear light consciousness; how, when the actual clear light consciousness has been aroused, one makes the transition to the "great union of training"; and, at the end of that process, how one makes the transition to the "great union beyond training"; how, in reliance upon retaining the clear light of sleep [in sleep yoga] and fortifying the ability to retain the energies in the central channel during the waking state, one brings the energies of the *rasana* and *lalana* channels into the central channel at the heart, and establishes the clear light consciousness by the stages of the four emptiness experiences; how, at the end of that process, one arises in the form of an illusory deity in the dream state; and so forth.

Thus although the illusory body and clear light doctrines are taught, some of the details are missing. However, nobody seems to have noticed or questioned this fact.

[As for the doctrine of sleep yoga,] there is the method of bringing the life-sustaining energies into the central channel, *avadhuti*, and retaining the clear light consciousness of sleep by means of controlling the energies. Alternatively, there is also the method of making firm the samadhi common to both the Hinayana and Mahayana during the waking state; then when going to sleep one places the mind in that state of samadhi and continues it in sleep. This can easily be mistaken for the tantric yoga of the clear light of sleep. These points are also not clearly discussed.

Likewise, a differentiation should be made between the yoga of retaining awareness during dreams by means of controlling the vital energies, and retaining awareness in dreams merely by means of conscious resolution.

As for the practice of blending with the clear light of death, there is the method implemented on the basis of controlling the vital energies; and alternatively there is the practice of developing concentration and applying this to the clear light of death. There is also the method that relies on intense resolution and reinforced familiarity. Likewise, there is the doctrine of how to arise as a Sambhogakaya buddha form in the bardo, the preparations for which must be made during the present time.

I have addressed these topics in detail in [my commentary to] the oral instruction tradition of the Arya Cycle of Guhyasamaja teachings [and therefore will not do so again here].

If one practices the yogas of sleep and dream by means of controlling the vital energies, the nature of the two suggests that one begin by fostering retention of the clear light of sleep. This can then be used as the basis of the dream yoga. This is pointed out in several of the manuals [on dream yoga].

If one is unable to bring the energies into the central channel, then during the daytime one should cultivate the resolution [to maintain conscious awareness during the dream state], and thus retain consciousness during dreams in that way. There is also the method of stabilizing concentration during the day, and then in sleep applying that samadhi in order to retain the clear light of sleep.

The above practice is termed "cultivating the clear light of sleep," but in fact includes the two [sleep and dream yogas]. The structure and order of the two is variable.

During the day one engages the outer and inner methods in order to cause the vital energies to enter, abide and dissolve within the central channel, thus generating the experiences of the famous four blisses and four emptinesses. When the innate bliss arises, one places awareness within it and engages the meditation of ecstasy and emptiness conjoined. Eventually one arises in the illusory body. After that, whatever appears in one's stream of experience is sealed with the stamp of ecstasy and emptiness. One meditates that all appearances arise as the mandala and mandala deities.

What is the principle behind working with the two extra chakras—the heart chakra in the practice of the clear light of sleep yoga, and the throat chakra in dream yoga?

[In the former case] one meditates upon the heart chakra because it is to the petals of the heart chakra that the vital energies naturally withdraw when one goes to sleep. Working with this chakra during the waking state brings familiarity with a technology that can be utilized in the sleep yogas, to be engaged when [during the process of entering into the sleep state] the subtle energies of the *rasana* and *lalana* channels naturally begin to withdraw into the central channel and the heart chakra. The force of the experience of the four emptinesses in general and the clear light emptiness in particular will be amplified. One fixes one's meditative absorption on this clear light of sleep as intensely as possible.

This training naturally augments one's ability to work with the vital energies during the waking state, as well as generally increasing the stability of the practice. Whether or not one has stabilized the ability to retain the clear light of sleep determines whether the power of traversing the path will be strong or weak.

Any proficiency achieved [in the yogas of sleep and dream] will bring great benefits at the time of death. Practitioners who have not managed to achieve supreme enlightenment in this life can attempt to do so then [by applying what was learned in the sleep and dream yogas]. As the moment of death approaches, they engage the unique methods for retaining the clear light of death, based on the degree of proficiency previously attained in the yogas of the clear light of sleep and of arising in the illusory body of the dream state. Familiarity with this technique causes the strength of one's illusory body practice to increase during the waking state, and that in turn supports one's practice of generating the illusory body of the dream state.

Should death arrive before supreme enlightenment has been attained, and one wishes to apply the yoga for enlightenment at the time of death, then [as the death process sets in] one engages the yogas of controlling the vital energies in order to recognize the clear light of the moment of death, using the same principles that were applied in the yoga of retaining the clear light of sleep. In this way one enters into the bardo experience, applies the techniques learned through the yoga of the illusory body of dreams, and generates the bardo body as the illusory body of the bardo.

Detailed instructions for this process [as given in the Six Yogas of Naropa] are not found elsewhere. These two oral instructions are undeceiving and are objects of supreme wonder and praise.

The manner of meditating on the individual paths

Now follows the explanation of how, as discussed earlier, one should meditate at auspicious times in both the sleeping and waking

states on the two principal teachings of the tantras, which are the
actual illusory body and clear light yogas. Other meditation techniques
[not taught in detail in the original tantric scriptures] abound in the
writings of the lineage masters of this tradition, and reference to some
of these will also be made.

Here there are two main topics: how to meditate on the illusory
body yogas; and how to meditate upon the clear light yogas.

How to meditate on the illusory body doctrine

The illusory body yogas are taught under three headings: how to
meditate on all appearances as illusory; how to meditate on dream
illusions; and how to meditate on the illusory nature of the bardo
experience.

How to meditate on all appearances as illusory

As explained earlier, during meditation sessions one conjoins
awareness of the view of profound emptiness, the ultimate nature,
together with the innate ecstasy. Then when one arises from the session the impact of the practice will carry over into the post-meditation period. Here [in times of non-formal sitting meditation] one
maintains awareness of the vision of emptiness, and recollects the
previous meditation on transforming all appearances into the mandala
and its deities. The strength of these two applications will cause all
appearances to arise as illusions, and as the supporting and supported
mandalas. No additional meditative techniques are required.

A practitioner who is unable to accomplish the above should, during meditation sessions, simply integrate with the [four] blisses produced through the tantric yogas. Then in the post-meditation periods, when the world and its inhabitants appear with an ambiance of
mundaneness, he or she should cultivate an awareness of the empty,
non-inherent nature of all phenomena.

Here a standard practice is to contemplate one's image reflected in
a mirror, to imagine that the reflected image is absorbed into oneself,
and then to think how one's body is like a reflected image. However,
this technique is really taught for those of small powers of practice,
and is not of great significance.[48]

One begins with the meditation on how the mundane world and
its inhabitants, while empty of inherent self-nature, manifest like illusions. When this becomes stable one causes the illusory appearances of world and inhabitants to arise as the pure supporting and

supported mandalas. One contemplates how all appearing phenomena are empty of having a self-nature, yet arise and are perceived as pure illusory mandala manifestations. There is also the tradition of reflecting an image of the mandala deity in a mirror and contemplating it. The image [is seen as] dissolving into oneself, and one meditates on oneself as having an illusory deity form. If the strength of the former meditation of this nature was made firm, then here no great effort will be required.

The tradition of *The Five Stages* speaks of how [during the empowerment ceremony] an image of Vajrasattva is reflected in a mirror and shown to disciples to demonstrate the nature of the illusory body. The guru first explains these two by means of metaphors and their meanings. If the disciple does not understand the words, then a visual image is shown. This is an extension of the generation stage visualizations, wherein a special mandala house is envisioned, various elements gathered, an image of the mandala deity reflected in a mirror, and one is instructed to meditate upon the reflected image. This practice is mentioned in the traditions of both Lama Marpa Lotsawa and Goe Lotsawa, and [as practiced today] is a blending of the two.

[The same text, *The Five Stages*, commenting on how] all phenomena are like illusions and like dreams, explains that the illusory nature is of two facets: the manner in which the manifest illusions point to ultimate reality, i.e., how things exist as mere momentary conventionals, and how this conventional existence eliminates the syndrome of apprehending things as having true existence; and secondly, the manner in which, even though things are empty of a self-nature, nonetheless they appear as illusions. The application here is the latter.

In this context there are two points to consider: the appearance itself; and the manner in which things are empty of existing in the mode of their appearance. We must appreciate both aspects. The nature of the appearance is not like that of a horn on a rabbit's head or the child of a barren woman [neither of which conventionally exist]. If there is no appearance, then we cannot speak of "empty of existing in the nature of its appearance." And if this does not arise in the mind, then the mind that can perceive the illusory nature of appearances will not arise.

One should understand all phenomena in the light of the simile of an illusion. For example, the illusory things created by a magician's spells, such as the horses and elephants that he causes to magically appear, are empty of actually being present [as living, breathing horses and elephants], yet still can be perceived by an audience of spectators. Their actual nature is utterly different from their ostensible presence.

This can be likened to the way in which we perceive the things of the world, such as persons and so forth. Although the objects of perception have forever utterly lacked a final self-nature or objective existence, nonetheless they indisputably appear with the nature of having real, inherent existence. The living beings who are perceived, such as humans and gods, and the forms, sounds and so forth that occur, are all in a state of continual transformation. And even though the living beings and other phenomena are without even the slightest inherent nature, nonetheless on the conventional level there are living beings who collect karma, there are the activities of seeing and hearing, and so forth. These things function conventionally on the basis of the laws of interdependence and causality.[49]

In this way conventional activity is accepted as omnipresent, and the extreme of nihilism is avoided. Conversely, because one appreciates the emptiness nature, the extreme of realism [or reification] is avoided.

This awareness of emptiness is simply an appreciation of the primordial non-inherently abiding nature of things. It is not a mental fabrication. Nor is it a partial emptiness that [is the nature of merely some phenomena and] does not pervade all objects of knowledge. By placing one's awareness on this final mode of being, all the forces that eliminate the syndrome of grasping at an "I" are strengthened.

That profound nature [i.e., emptiness] is not an inaccessible object of awareness. By ascertaining the pure view of emptiness and acquiring familiarity with meditation upon that quintessential aspect of being, it arises as an object of the mind. Thus it is not an emptiness, as some would say, that cannot be engaged at the time of practice, nor an emptiness that cannot be perceived or realized.

In brief, one examines one's person, the apprehender of an "I," and asks whether this "final nature" that appears exists as either one with or separate from the body-mind aggregates. One discovers that it does not even slightly exist in either place. Thus the living beings are seen to utterly lack true existence. One makes one's experience of this awareness firm. This is the training on the emptiness side of things.

As for the training on the conventional side, i.e., that of interdependent co-existence, here one turns the mind's awareness to how on the functional level all things indisputably appear as existing. Living beings manifest as objects of conventional perception, as collectors of karma, and as experiencers of the results of karma. We should cultivate a definite realization of how, although having no self-nature, all phenomena conventionally function with validity according to the laws of interdependent arising.

Whenever these two levels of being seem contradictory, use the simile of an image reflected in a mirror to appreciate their non-contradictory nature. Contemplate how the reflected image of a face, including the eyes and so forth, are empty of existing in the manner of their appearance. Based on the presence of an image to be reflected, as well as the mirror and so forth, the reflection is created. When one takes away the supporting conditions, such as either the face or the mirror, the image disappears. The two [emptiness nature and appearing nature] have a commonly shared base.

Therefore there is not a single particle within living beings to represent a final self; yet living beings collect karmic seeds, experience the results, and take rebirths according to their previously collected karmic seeds and the presence of the spiritual distortions within themselves. One must appreciate the non-contradictory nature [of emptiness and relativity] in this way.

When one has achieved stability in this realization one extends it to the world, which is seen as the mandala; and to living beings, who are seen as tantric deities. Then one trains in the method of the playful view that dwells within ecstasy and emptiness conjoined.

By practicing in this way, all appearances become mandala and deities. These in turn appear as illusions, and the illusions arise as great ecstasy. These are the three stages of the process.

During meditation sessions one invokes the great ecstasy, uses this as the driving force in the focus upon the view of emptiness, and then rests single-pointedly within that absorption of beyond-conceptuality mind. Between sessions one cultivates the awareness of how emptiness and conventional interdependent existence complement one another.

In this way the two [formal sessions and between-session trainings] are applied in rotation as complementary to and supportive of one another.

How to meditate on dream illusions

This involves four trainings: learning to retain [conscious presence during] dreams; controlling and increasing dreams; overcoming fear and training in the illusory nature of dreams; and meditating upon the suchness of dreams.

Learning to retain [conscious presence during] dreams

Conscious presence can be retained during dreams by either of two methods.

In the first of these, which involves working with the vital energies, one gathers the vital energies into the central channel during the waking state and dissolves them, inducing the experiences of the four emptinesses [i.e., appearance, proximity, proximate attainment and clear light]. The manner of the application is that in the process of first retaining the clear light of sleep one cultivates awareness of the four emptinesses of sleep. After that, when dreams occur one recognizes them as such. When awareness of the four emptinesses of sleep is present, no other technique for retention of awareness in dreams is required.

The second method involves conscious resolution. If one is not able to succeed in the above method [of controlling the subtle energies as the means of working with the dream state], then during the waking state one should cultivate a strong resolution to retain conscious awareness in the dream state. In addition, one meditates on the chakras, especially that at the throat.

The first of the above two techniques is the principal method of retaining dreams as taught exclusively in highest yoga tantra. The second is shared in common with other ways.

In the tradition of Lama Tsur (Tib. *'Tshur gyi lugs*), the dream retention yoga is accomplished in conjunction with meditating on the heart chakra. The tradition of Lama Mey (Tib. *Mes kyi lugs*) recommends instead working with the throat chakra. There are these two explanations.

Some manuals comment that the meditations on the heart chakra are associated with the yoga of the clear light of sleep, and those on the throat chakra are associated with dream yoga. However, if the dream yoga is being implemented by means of controlling the vital energies, then first one must apply the technology for recognizing the four emptinesses of the moment of sleep; this is accomplished by working with the heart chakra.

On the other hand, if one does not have the ability to recognize the experiences of the four emptinesses as a means of retaining conscious awareness in dreams, and consequently the yoga is being implemented solely on the basis of resolution, then one meditates on the throat chakra.

Does this explanation of how the throat chakra is linked to retaining dreams mean that the throat chakra is only engaged when the method is that of conscious resolution?

[No. For example,] in the method of retaining dreams by means of controlling the vital energies, the throat chakra can be visualized at the time of going to sleep in order to bring the energies to this chakra and give rise to the experience of the four emptinesses there. However, if previously the energies had not been collected at the heart chakra then they will not collect now at the throat chakra. Because an experience of the four emptinesses like that induced by dissolving the energies at the heart will not arise at other sites, in the dream yogas one mainly meditates on the heart chakra at the time of going to sleep.

Through meditating on the chakras at the throat, forehead and so forth when going to sleep one causes the energies that had gathered at the heart to become somewhat diffused. This has the effect of making one's sleep less deep, and thus of rendering it easier to retain conscious awareness [during dreams]. Moreover, familiarity with meditation at the throat chakra when going to sleep causes one's dreams to last longer.

If in the process of the dream yoga one wishes to extend the duration of one's dreams, then before going to sleep one meditates on the throat chakra as before. As soon as the mind holds to it for a moment, then within the dream sphere one engages in whatever spiritual exercises are appropriate. Thus the throat chakra here becomes instrumental in the dream yoga technology.

There is a point that should be made on the practice of retaining conscious awareness in the dream state by means of cultivating resolution. In general, even people who are not trained sometimes can experience a clear dream and retain awareness in it. Therefore it is not only through the path of meditation on retaining dream awareness that the ability occurs. For example, if someone concentrates strongly on a particular activity all day, then at night he may dream of it, and may even be aware of that dream. Consequently if we make some effort during the daytime to cultivate a strong resolution to recognize and remember our dreams, and we make this resolution strong and continuous throughout the day, then at night dreams will certainly arise and one will probably be able to retain them. This level of the practice is not difficult to accomplish.

Should dreams fail to occur, however, it will not be possible to engage in the dream yogas. Dreams are required as the basis. Moreover, even if one does experience dreams it will not be easy to recognize them if they are unclear. One needs to achieve clarity in them. For a dream to fit this description, one should be able to describe it in detail to others upon waking.

In the beginning of practice, clear dreams are necessary. To achieve this it may be necessary to dwell in solitary retreat in order to achieve clear dreaming, for solitude enhances mental clarity. Then in the early morning, when consciousness is especially clear, it will become easy to retain the dreams.

In this way during the daytime one generates strong instincts through application of resolution. These must be aroused during the dream state and used to induce a clear awareness in dreams. To accomplish this, one must practice during the daytime.

Here the oral tradition suggests that this is best effected by meditating during the day on the chakras at the throat and forehead, using the radiant visualizations as described. The mind should first be clarified by means of the breathing exercises that unite the vital energies.

If one understands these guidelines as presented in the oral tradition, one will become increasingly skilled in generating the appropriate experiences. Otherwise [if one doesn't understand the guidelines], only a small result will be achieved. Here the instructions are much the same in the different oral traditions.

In the practice of retaining dreams it is useful to meditate upon oneself as the mandala deity, and also to meditate upon the guru and practice devotion to him or her. Offer prayers that one may experience many dreams, that the dreams may be clear and auspicious, that one may retain awareness in one's dreams, and that one may effectively engage the special applications in the dream state. One also offers prayers that unconducive conditions to these ends may not arise, and that every conducive condition may become manifest. For this one makes *torma* offerings to the mandala deities and protectors, requests their enlightened activity, and establishes the basis of the practice.

Thus during the day, one continually cultivates the strong resolution, combining this with the practice of repeating to oneself that whatever appears is like a dream occurrence and should be recognized as a dream. Then when dreams occur, one consciously recognizes and retains awareness during them, and thus becomes able to implement the dream yoga practices. Directing one's thoughts in this way, one makes stable the throwing force of resolution. Then when clear dreams arise, one will be able to recognize and retain awareness of them. This method in itself is sufficient.

There are three instructions on how to apply the forceful methods at night as taught in the oral tradition.

In the first of these, one places the mind on the mantric syllable at the throat chakra. Then before going to sleep one generates the vision of oneself as the mandala deity, with one's guru seated above one's head, and offers prayers to the guru inseparable from the mandala deity. Inside the central channel at the throat chakra one visualizes a small red four-petalled lotus, with either a small red mantric syllable of *AH* or *OM* standing upon it. This is in nature the vajra speech, the communicative power of enlightenment. One maintains this visualization with clarity, not allowing the mind to lose it, and falls asleep within the sphere of retaining it.

Some oral traditions suggest that five mantric syllables be visualized—*OM, AH, NU, TA,* and *RA*—with one at the center and the other four around it. One meditates upon these successively. Others suggest that one simply visualize the red syllable *AH* in the center of the lotus. Thus there are two alternative traditions.

The scripture *The Victorious Non-Duality Tantra* (Skt. *Advaya vijaya tantra*) comments that one may visualize the mantric syllables *OM, AH, NU, TA* and *RA* standing in a circle on a four-petalled lotus, but adds that this does not bring any extra power to the practice [and therefore visualizing a simple *OM* in the center will suffice].

Many tantric texts, including *The Sambhuta Tantra*, recommend the syllable *OM*. However, it is not inappropriate instead to use the mantric syllable *AH*. The important thing, whichever mantric syllable is used, is that it is visualized inside the central channel at the center of the throat chakra, and that one holds awareness on that spot. If one does this and still one cannot retain the dreams, then repeat the earlier exercises.

Should one still be unable to retain the dream, then one should meditate on the drop in the chakra at the forehead. Now, sleep is usually very thick during the period of the very early morning, and consequently it is very difficult to retain dreams at that time. Sleep is lightest following the period of dawn until after the sun has arisen from the eastern mountains. Consequently it is easier to retain one's dreams at that time.

One meditates on guru yoga and offers prayers that the dream yogas may be accomplished. Next one generates a strong resolution as before, and creates the vision of oneself as the mandala deity. Then place the mind on the radiant white drop, the size of a mustard seed, located between the eyebrows. Perform the vase breathing technique seven times, and go back to sleep.

Here do not visualize the drop as being excessively bright, for this may result in not being able to go back to sleep, or in sleeping only a little while and then awakening. Visualize the drop as being somewhat less bright.

Some teachers say that if one first places the mind at the syllable at the throat chakra one will not be able to go back to sleep, and that therefore one should first visualize the white drop at the forehead chakra. This isn't particularly sensible. The throat chakra is the site from which dreams are generated, and the forehead chakra, that associated with the waking state. In effect what they are saying is that meditating on the site associated with dreams will hinder sleep, yet meditating on the site associated with the waking state will not.

If one performs the above practice at the throat chakra at dusk or after dawn and still one is not able to retain one's dreams, this indicates that the practitioner is a person who naturally sleeps very deeply. To somewhat lighten the nature of sleep one should place the mind on the crown chakra.

If in turn this causes one to be unable to sleep, or to sleep fitfully, then concentrate instead on the drop at the secret place. Here during the daytime one cultivates the resolution described earlier, and works with the chakra at the tip of the jewel. Before going to sleep one visualizes there a dark drop, and unites the vital energies twenty-one times [through vase breathing]. Within that sphere, and without letting the mind stray, one drops off to sleep.

Sometimes working with the upper sites causes one's sleep to become too light. If this occurs, one should keep in mind that the chakra at the jewel is also associated with the sleep state, and therefore placing the mind on it will affect the depth of one's sleep. One must know how to work with the different chakras at dusk and dawn in this way in order to bring the elements [i.e., the drops within the chakras] into balance.

Some people apply themselves to these methods but still cannot gain the ability to work with dreams. They may persist in the method for months or years, and even then not produce the desired results. These beings must rely upon the method of first cultivating the inner heat, bringing the vital energies into the central channels, causing these to abide and dissolve, and meditating on the innate wisdom. If they cannot generate the experience of the innate wisdom, they will not be able to retain the clear light of sleep. And without retaining the clear light of sleep through control of the vital energies they will not be able to retain awareness in dreams.

Thus if prolonged effort at retaining dreams through cultivating the power of resolution does not produce the desired results, one should not regard the situation as impossible. Instead one should remember that the inner heat practice is the foundation of this path and return to it. In fact the cultivation of resolution is really intended as an aid, and not as the principal technique in dream yoga. To bypass the method of the inner heat and instead to rely solely upon cultivating the power of resolution is like throwing away the trunk of the tree and keeping only the branches.

Controlling and increasing dreams

The practice of controlling the contents of illusory dreams is of two types.

The first of these is the control of worldly contents. Here one can engage in various transformative exercises, such as consciously initiating a particular dream pattern, or else transforming the nature of the dream altogether. Alternatively, one can project oneself on the rays of the sun or moon to a celestial realm, such as the Thirty-Three Heaven, or to a faraway human realm, and see what is there. One trains in these various activities, such as going to places, flying through the sky, and so forth.

The second type of this practice involves controlling the contents of beyond-the-world dreams. This involves consciously projecting oneself in the dream state to the various buddhafields, such as

Sukhavati, Tushita, Akanishta, and so forth, and while there meeting with the buddhas and bodhisattvas, venerating them, listening to their teachings, and so forth.

When these techniques are being implemented by means of controlling the vital energies, then one conjoins the principles of energy control with those of generating strong resolution. This renders the practice more easily accomplished. Those who do not have the power of energy control should familiarize themselves with the exercise of cultivating resolution.

These two applications are used for perceiving the pure dimensions of the world and its inhabitants. In fact the "pure realms" experienced [by those on initial stages] are mere reflections of the real thing. It is not that easy to experience the actual pure dimensions.

As for prophecies received during such experiences, although certain prophecies of future happenings may be true, mostly they will not be. When the dream visions are related to past events [such as one's past lives], one should apply the yogic techniques for increasing reliability, such as certain methods of application during the dream process, particular energy control techniques, and so forth.

As for the exercise of "increasing in dreams," this refers to increasing the number of whatever appears in the dream: whether sentient beings such as humans or animals, or inanimate objects such as a pillar or a vase. One multiplies the object from one to two, from two to four, and so forth, until hundreds and even thousands of the object appear.

Overcoming fear and training in the illusory nature of dreams

During the dreaming process whenever anything of a threatening or traumatic nature occurs, such as drowning in water or being burned by fire, recognize the dream as a dream and ask yourself, "How can dream water or dream fire possibly harm me?" Make yourself jump or fall into the water or fire in the dream.

The method of training in the illusory nature of dreams entails that we take one of the dream objects, such as a vase or the like, and remind ourselves that, even though this object is appearing in the dream, nonetheless it is empty of the nature of its appearance. Recognize dream objects as dream objects.

However, merely this awareness will not necessarily mean that the non-inherent nature of dream objects is appreciated. For example, when we look at the image in a mirror during the waking state we may be aware of the empty nature of the image [in the sense that it is not the actual object being reflected]; but we will not necessarily have perceived its "suchness" nature.

When one fails to recognize the dream as a dream, the situation is like that of a young infant who looks at his own reflection in a mirror and thinks it to be a real person. Seeing a dream as a dream is like the adult who looks at his image in a mirror, and perceives that although the face appears in the mirror, nonetheless it is empty of possessing any actual human being.

We should take the example of how a reflected image is empty of being what it appears to be, and apply this to every phenomenon in order to understand how each is empty of having an inherent self-nature that exists from its own side. Similarly with recognizing the dream as a dream, one takes the above example [of how, like the reflected image, the dream is empty of existing in the nature of its appearance] and applies this to how all phenomena are empty of possessing even the tiniest bit of true existence. One should understand exactly how strong the presence of the syndrome of grasping at a self-nature is, and understand the strength of the pure reasoning required to undermine it.

On the basis of that understanding one transforms the dream world and its inhabitants into the supporting and supported mandala [i.e., residence and deities]. One meditates on how all these appearances are empty of a true self-nature, yet manifest as illusions. Cultivate the vision of how all phenomena are a drama of ecstasy and void.

These meditations are also to be applied during the waking state.

Meditating upon suchness in dreams

This is to be differentiated from the practice of clear light yoga. Here one begins by meditating upon oneself in the luminous appearance of the mandala deity, the mantric syllable *HUM* at one's heart radiating with a great profusion of light. This [light] melts the animate and inanimate dream objects [into light], which is drawn into the *HUM*. One's body then also melts into light, from the head downward and feet upward, and is absorbed into the *HUM*. The *HUM* then melts into unapprehendable clear light. One rests the mind unwaveringly within this light.

It is easier to absorb the appearance of dream objects into light than it is to absorb the energies from the objects that appear to the mind during the waking state. However, if at that time [of engaging dream yoga] one applies the technologies for absorbing certain of the coarse energies and they come to the heart chakra, then dreams will not arise and instead one will enter into deep sleep.

As a remedy, cultivate recognition of the four emptinesses [i.e., the four stages of entering into the sleep state]. If this does not succeed with the first few attempts, then one persists until eventually the ability to clearly discern these "four emptinesses of sleep" is achieved.

To accomplish stability in these processes of the absorptions and the emptinesses, during the daytime one enhances the practice through the meditations on uniting the energies [i.e., the vase breathing technique], and so forth. Then at night when first going to sleep one attempts to recognize the stages of absorption and the four emptinesses of sleep.

If this does not work, then after the dreams have commenced one should apply the methods discussed earlier. The force to recognize them should thus be aroused.

How to meditate on the illusory nature of the bardo experience

This yoga is taught under two headings: a discussion of the underlying philosophy of the bardo experience; and a discussion of the stages of the bardo yoga practice.

The underlying philosophy of the bardo experience

The moment when death arrests the life force, and the moment when the bardo experience is produced: these two arise like the up and down movements of a weight scale.

One is instantly born into the bardo with a body complete in all sensory powers. In shape it resembles that of the incarnation to be taken, and it possesses great karmic powers of miraculous physical ability. With the exception of the place of future rebirth, it can travel anywhere without impediment, and can pass freely through solid matter.[50]

The life span of this bardo body is a maximum of seven days, yet even this length is not definite. At the end of this period it ceases; and, if one has not taken rebirth into the world, then another bardo body appears. Again, if one does not find conditions for rebirth within the seven days of its life span, then it dies, and one gets a third bardo body. In this way one can repeat the cycle seven times, making a total of forty-nine bardo days. After that one will certainly have to take rebirth.

One receives a sign indicating which of the four types of birth one is attracted to: miraculous birth, birth by heat and moisture, birth from an egg, or birth from a womb. In the first situation, one is attracted to the place of the rebirth. If the birth indicated is by heat and moisture, one is attracted to the smells, tastes, and so forth of the place. When the birth is to be by egg or from a womb, one develops lust and aversion at the vision of the future parents having actual intercourse or seeming intercourse.

Moreover, when one is unfolding toward rebirth as a female, lust arises toward the father and aversion toward the mother. Conversely, if one is unfolding toward rebirth as a male, lust for the mother arises, and aversion for the father.

For some it is their aversion to a place that will bring them to take rebirth in it.

Those in the bardo who are experiencing the effects of past negative karmic deeds experience a dark vision, like that of a night sky with no stars. Those of positive karmic disposition experience a clear and radiant vision, like that of a white woolen cloth, or like a night sky filled with moonlight.

When the bardo experience is leading to a rebirth in one of the hell realms, one's bodily color resembles a burned tree stump. When it is leading to the animal realms, one's color is like that of smoke. When it is leading to the world of ghosts, one's body is a color like that of water; and when the bardo is leading to rebirth in the human or sensual god realms, it is a golden color. The bardo being who is destined for the form realms is white in color. This is related in *The Sutra on Entering into the Womb* (Skt. *Garbha vakranti sutra*).

This same sutra states,

> Those beings who [die in and thus] leave the formless realms do experience a bardo. However, beings who die in the two lower realms [i.e., the *kamadhatu* and *rupadhatu*] and are destined for birth in the formless realms experience no bardo whatsoever. Immediately after leaving their old bodies they take rebirth in the formless realm, with the aggregates [i.e., the body-mind base] of that formless world.

Others say that there is no bardo associated with the formless realms, because the formless realms have no upper or lower boundaries. This is their own idea [and there is no scriptural basis for the doctrine].

The Treasury of Abhidharma (Skt. *Abhidharma kosha*) states, "...having the form of the future incarnation." Thus the Abhidharma literature suggests that the form of one's body in the bardo resembles that of the future existence.

Not understanding this passage, some teachers have said that the form resembles that of the previous life, and that one's companions and so forth of that life manifest. Others have quoted *The Compendium of Abhidharma* (Skt. *Abhidharma samucchaya*), wherein it is said, "The face and body resemble those of the future life." Having seen this passage, they state that one's form in the bardo is that of one's future incarnation, and that one's friends of that incarnation will also manifest [in the bardo experience].[51]

Still others speak of a bardo body that is a blending of the two above ideas of past and future forms. Here it is said that during the first three and a half days [of each seven-day cycle], one has the form and world vision of the previous life, and during the last three and a half days, the form and vision of the future life. After the three-and-a-half day period one experiences the awareness that one has died and is in the bardo. Such is their theory; but no authoritative scriptural source whatsoever for it is ever given, nor is it supported particularly well by reason. Thus it is mere speculation.

The etymology of the term "bardo" is given in *A Treasury of Abhidharma*,

> We die in this world, and later take rebirth;
> Between these two is "the bardo world."

Thus the sense is that the bardo world is experienced from the moment of our death until rebirth takes place. Hence it is an "in-between realm." There is nothing other than life, death and the bardo, or "state in-between"; thus it is simply called "the in-between of becoming," or "the in-between realm." This is the sense of the above Abhidharma passage.

However, in this tradition [i.e., that of the Six Yogas] we see three "bardo states" being mentioned.[52] Firstly, there is "the bardo between birth and death," which refers to the [waking-state] period from our birth to our death, including the present moment. Secondly, there is "the dream bardo," which is the period between when we go to sleep until we wake up. Thirdly, the time from death until rebirth is known as "the bardo realm," or "the bardo of becoming."

What is the sense of this mode of categorizing existential experience?

Here the Arya Cycle of the Guhyasamaja tradition speaks of how the experience of the four emptinesses [of appearance, proximity, proximate attainment and clear light] gives rise to the clear light. This is experienced much the same way as the clear light of death is experienced after the dissolution of bodily processes is complete. The yogi then produces the illusory body [by means of the four emptinesses and blisses mentioned above]; this is similar to how the bardo body is produced [after the clear light of death]. This [i.e., the illusory body] becomes the subtle Sambhogakaya, which takes upon itself a coarse Nirmanakaya form, much in the same way that the bardo body takes rebirth with a worldly form.

Those beings who do not possess yogic abilities will experience these three occasions as ordinary birth, death and bardo. However, yogis holding the oral tradition teachings know how to take the three kayas at the time of the path [i.e., the ordinary dimensions of these three] and transform them into the three kayas at the time of the result [i.e., in buddhahood]. Appreciating the similarities and connections between the three occasions [birth, death and bardo] and three kayas, during both occasions of path and result, the name "the three occasions for spiritual practice" is applied to the basis of the three kayas on these three occasions, and the name "the three kayas" is also applied to the three events as the basis. I have discussed these ideas in detail elsewhere.

Suffice it to say here that when during the waking state we meditate upon producing the illusory body, this is similar to the manner in which the bardo body arises; therefore the name "bardo" is sometimes applied to this occasion. Similarly, when we enter into the clear light of the moment of sleep and then pass into the dream state, the illusory dream body that arises is similar in nature to the bardo body; this is the reason for using the expression "the dream bardo." And because when special [i.e., highly trained] beings pass through the stage of the clear light of death and enter into the bardo they apply the technology for manifesting [the bardo body as] a Sambhogakaya form, this experience is also termed a "bardo."

Thus in this tradition we see these three predominant usages of the term "bardo." However, those who understand correctly the context of the application are rare. The sense is that the three occasions of the basis [i.e., birth, death and bardo] are to be transformed into occasions for manifestation of the three kayas. The meaning is that the two sets of three are to be blended.

In brief, the above description leads to there being talk of three "illusory bodies": the illusory body of the waking state; that of the

illusory dream body; and the illusory body which is produced in the
bardo. These three are linked to the three bardos of the [three] basic
occasions [waking state, dreams and bardo].

How do we proceed in the training of these three bardos?

Here during the waking state one practices meditation on the inner heat, thus causing the vital energies to enter into the central channel, and to abide and dissolve. Through the force of this experience
one induces the experiences of the four emptinesses, four blisses, and
the clear light consciousness. The experience is like that of the time of
death, when the vital energies and consciousnesses naturally withdraw from the body into the central channel and the clear light of
death manifests.

The meditations on the three clear light consciousnesses—the clear
light experienced through yogic endeavor in the waking state, the
clear light of sleep, and the clear light of the moment of death—are
similar in that all three require that one understand the process of
dissolving the vital energies and consciousnesses into the central channel just as at the moment of death, and how thus to induce the experience of the four emptinesses and four blisses.

If one understands these three sets of three processes, then in the
waking state application the subtle illusory body can take the form of
a coarse Nirmanakaya. Also, the dream yoga can be used in the gap
at the end of dreams and before waking up to cause the subtle
Sambhogakaya [generated in dream yoga] to take a coarse Nirmanakaya. Similarly, after the moment of the clear light of death has passed
and one enters the bardo, the same technique can be used to transform the bardo body into a Sambhogakaya form; and that in turn can
be used to take a coarse Nirmanakaya form.

This process is sophisticated, and one should attempt to get a clear
comprehension of it. If one can gain insight into the basic principles
at work in the dissolutions, then the three blendings—the clear light
of death with the Dharmakaya, the bardo body with the Sambhogakaya, and the rebirth body with the Nirmanakaya—can be
accomplished.

In brief, the dynamics of these three peerless processes—or, if each
of the three is spoken of as threefold, then the nine processes—should
be understood well.

Mistaking the basic thrust of this doctrine, some teachers apply
the concept of the three blendings quite differently, stating that one
blends passion with the third empowerment, confusion with the clear

light, and aversion with the illusory body. However, although it is true that one does adopt the path of passion when actually receiving the third initiation, this empowerment is in fact just a preliminary [in the overall tantric training], which one needs in order to take up the meditations and yogas of the generation and completion stages of tantric application. Now, during the generation stage yoga there is no technique for these blendings; and even though this technology is taught in the completion stage yogas, it is not associated with the above phase of practice.

Extending the doctrine that when the bardo being enters the womb of its new rebirth it experiences lust for the parent of the opposite sex and aversion toward the parent of the same sex [as the being it will be in its next lifetime], some lamas have stated that one should blend aversion with the illusory body. They pronounce this based on the above doctrine, and with no other supporting reason. However, they do not elucidate how this is relevant to the all-important illusory body yoga of the waking state, or to the blending of the illusory body of dreams. [Of the three illusory body yogas, i.e., those of waking state, dreams and bardo,] here it seems that these teachers are discarding the first two very important types of illusory body yoga in favor of the third. In addition, this approach doesn't address the problem of how, once the clear light of the moment of death has passed and one enters into the bardo, the bardo body is blended with the illusory body dynamic [to produce the Sambhogakaya]. Moreover, the association made with aversion is rather random; for example, at the time of entering the womb the bardo being is also said to generate lust [for the parent of the opposite sex], so the illusory body yoga could just as validly be linked with passion. Thus the concept doesn't seem particularly useful.

Another quaint idea one sometimes sees proposes that because lust is strong in life, one should then blend lust with the bardo of birth to death; [because confusion is strong in dreams,] one should blend confusion with the bardo of dreams; and [because aversion is strong in the bardo,] one should blend aversion with the bardo of becoming [between death and rebirth]. [In this way one blends the three root klesha, or emotional and perceptual distortions, with the three bardos.] This also is not a particularly useful hypothesis, for the reasons stated above. In particular, it does not account for the passage in the tantric scriptures that states, "In the space between sleep and dream lies confusion, in nature the Dharmakaya." As this quotation indicates, on going to sleep and before entering dreams one should recognize and retain the experience of the clear light of sleep. They accept the above quotation as valid and link it to blending confusion and dreams, whereas the "confusion" in the passage actually refers to the clear light experience. Thus the passage they use to support their idea in fact contradicts what they are trying to say.

Some people claim that in some remote corner of Marpa's oral instructions there is the teaching that one should blend lust with non-ejaculation yoga, aversion with the illusory body yoga, and confusion with the clear light yoga. The first two of these statements are unconvincing.

Also, some lamas speak of the three "blendings" as follows. The meditations on the two yogic stages [i.e., generation and completion stage] are to be blended with the bardo of birth and death; after cultivating that process, the dream bardo is to be blended with confusion and the clear light, and brought into the two tantric stages in that way; and, thirdly, the bardo of becoming is to be blended with aversion and *dharmata* [i.e., the ultimate nature of things], and thus brought into the two tantric stages. This is the interpretation they give to "the three blendings." Although this is said, I fail to see any real sense in it.

There is also a discussion of further sub-dividing the three bodies of the three bardo states, until we get fifteen bardos. As this is rather simplistic, I will not write of it here.

The stages of the bardo yoga practice

This is discussed under two headings: the types of beings who can practice in the bardo; and the nature of the training.

The types of beings who can practice in the bardo

It is said that there are three levels of beings who can practice in the bardo: best, medium and least.

The qualities of the first of these are mentioned in tantric scriptures such as *The Book of Manjushri's Direct Instructions* (Skt. *Manjushri mukhagama*), *A Compendium of Tantric Experiences* (Skt. *Charya melapaka pradipa*), and *The Clear Lamp* (Skt. *Pradipoddyotana*), wherein it is said that the best practitioner takes the bardo body that appears at the end of the dying process and transforms it into a Sambhogakaya, and on that basis accomplishes enlightenment in the bardo.

Therefore there is the saying from some Tibetan lama-scholars of old that states, "The lazy attain enlightenment in the bardo." Actually, they are not really that lazy. It is simply that they did not accomplish all the conditions of enlightenment during their lifetime, but came close enough so that enlightenment could be attained in the bardo. Thus they are only called "lazy" from one particular perspective.

How deep must be the state of realization accomplished in this lifetime in order for one to qualify as the "best bardo practitioner"?

One must have completed the realizations of the generation stage yogas and then, in the completion stage yogas, must have mastered the technique of directing the vital energies into the central channel and causing them to abide and dissolve, thus generating the experiences of the four blisses and four emptinesses, together with the according primordial wisdoms. Thus they must have almost reached the stage of manifesting the actual illusory body in their meditations.

The mark of medium practitioners is that they are able to bring the vital energies into the central channel and dissolve them, thus generating the four emptinesses. Based on that ability they gain the power to achieve the blending of the clear light of sleep [during their lifetime]. This is a highly praised accomplishment, for through the power of that energy control they are able to engage the blending of the emptiness of the clear light of death. Thus if during their lifetime they are able to blend with the emptiness of deep sleep, then at death they will be able to blend with the clear light of death. If even in very deep sleep they are able to retain the clear light of sleep, this is an excellent sign.

As for the least qualification for practicing the bardo yoga, here the trainee must have received the empowerments, be stable in guarding the tantric commitments, have made some progress in the generation stage yogas, and have cultivated some familiarity with the completion stage yogas.

Then when the time of death arrives, he or she maintains awareness as the signs of the dissolution process occur, beginning with the earth energies dissolving into those of water, and so forth, up to the emergence of the clear light of death. Knowledgeable of this process, he or she observes it closely, an ability acquired by having cultivated fluency in the oral tradition teachings on the process. The technique is similar to the manner in which the dream yoga is accomplished by means of resolution. He or she is unable to recognize and retain the clear light of death by means of the energy control yogas, and so engages in the bardo yogas on the strength of previous familiarity with the oral tradition teachings.

Alternatively, for those who are not qualified in this way, but who have achieved some meditative stability, then as the moment of death draws near they should engage in their samadhi and make the stream of it strong, meditating in accordance with the way they practiced during their lifetime. The strength of this will then carry over into the bardo. If during this crucial experience that positive mind can be recollected, it will have a beneficial impact on the process of dying and the bardo. However, this is a quite ordinary samadhi application.

The nature of the training

The best of the three types of practitioners are said to accomplish buddhahood in the bardo. They were unable to do so during their actual lifetime, but during the death process are able to recognize the manifestation of the clear light and apply the according technology.

There is the popular saying, "One achieves enlightenment on first entering into the bardo." This isn't particularly meaningful, and contradicts many authoritative tantric scriptures. The moment of first entering the bardo refers to the culmination of the clear light experience. The clear light vision is actually classified as belonging to this life [and not the bardo]. Moreover, no authoritative tantric scriptures speak of enlightenment being achieved at that moment.

To attain the Dharmakaya for the first time one must rely upon a suitable body-base. Otherwise the established doctrines on the process are contradicted. The body-base present at that moment [i.e., the first moment of the bardo] could not manifest the marks and signs of the accomplishment states of "great union of training" and "great union beyond training."

Thus the expression "blend the clear light of death with the Dharmakaya" actually refers to recognizing the clear light of death and blending it with a sense of something approximating the Dharmakaya. The name "Dharmakaya" is given to this phenomenon, but it is not the actual Dharmakaya.

The yogi must pass through the death process and emerge with a bardo body. But even then merely recognizing the bardo and applying simple yogas on the basis of that [ordinary bardo body] will not produce the supreme accomplishment of buddhahood.

Here the best type of practitioner must recognize the nature of the bardo body, and then control the most subtle aspects of energy and mind in order to transform it into a Sambhogakaya form. Elsewhere [I have] discussed in detail the methods of doing this.

Those who belong to the category of the two types of "less-qualified practitioners" should attempt to bring the mind into a state of clarity as the moment of death approaches. In their thoughts they dedicate all their worldly possessions to worthy receivers and sources of merit. Thus they sever all conditions of attachment. They should consciously acknowledge to themselves any transgressions of their practice guidelines that occurred during their lifetime, as well as any general spiritual failings, and then purify these and renew their spiritual precepts. In this way they squarely face the thought of impending death without any attachments or fears.

Those familiar with the oral tradition teachings on the stages of dying and the nature of the bardo offer prayers and cultivate the resolution to remember the guidelines of advice during the dying and bardo experiences, and generate joy like a child returning to its parents' house. As the moment of death approaches they generate the vision of self-identification with the mandala deity, visualizing the gurus and the assembly of enlightenment deities in the space in front, offering them devotions, and sending forth prayers for inspiration and blessings for success in applying the yogas of blending with the clear light at the moment of death, and thereafter blending with the illusory bardo body.

The second type of practitioner, prior to the arising of the signs of death that occur in the dying process, applies whatever abilities he or she possesses in order to cause the energies to enter the central channel and give rise to the experience of the four emptinesses. At the conclusion of that phase he or she applies the special methods for arising as a mandala deity, of recognizing the four emptinesses of entering into sleep, and applying the same technology as was used for generating the illusory body of dreams. He or she repeats these exercises many times [prior to the onset of the dying process], and then observes for the signs of elemental dissolution that precede the experience of death. This involves the twenty states of dissolution that occur during the dying process prior to the experience of the clear light of death.

In brief this process is as follows.

First the earth element dissolves into the water element. The external sign is that one loses the ability to move one's limbs or control the body, and has an appearance of total relaxation. The thought arises, "My body is sinking into the earth," and there is an urge to call for someone to pull one up. The inner sign is a vision having a mirage-like quality.

Next the water element dissolves into the fire element. The external sign is dryness of mouth and nose, and a shrivelling of the tongue. The inner sign is a vision as though of smoke.

The fire element now dissolves into the air element. The external sign is that one's body heat begins to drop, withdrawing from the extremities [toward the heart]. The inner sign is a vision like that of seeing many fireflies.

The air element of conceptual thought dissolves into mind. Here the vital energies that support conceptual thought dissolve into consciousness. The external sign is that a long breath is exhaled, and the body seems unable to inhale. Even if one can inhale, one does so shallowly yet heavily. The inner sign is a vision of a light resembling that of a butterlamp undisturbed by wind movement.

After this the first emptiness occurs, known simply as "emptiness." This is the experience of the vision known as "appearance." The inner sign is of whiteness, like seeing moonlight in a cloudless sky.

The consciousness of "appearance" then dissolves into the second emptiness, known as "very empty." This is the experience of the vision known as "proximity." The inner vision is of a yellowish red light, like that of the light at sunrise.

This dissolves into the third emptiness, "the great emptiness," which is linked to the experience of the vision known as "proximate attainment." The inner vision is of utter darkness, like that of a night sky pervaded by thick darkness. The person has a sensation of swooning, and loses consciousness.

After this the person emerges from the darkness and the state of mindlessness, and arises into the experience of "utter emptiness," also termed "the clear light." The vision is of a color like the blending of the lights of sun and moon in a sky free from all darkness, like the clear sky at early dawn. This is the clear light that is the actual basis.

In this way one experiences the three emptinesses, together with the "emptiness" of the clear light consciousness.

In the stages of experiencing the three emptinesses and the clear light emptiness, first there are the external signs of the dissolution of the elements: the visions as though of a mirage, of smoke, of fireflies, of the light of a butterlamp, and of a cloudless sky. The signs of the inner dissolutions are those of whiteness, redness, blackness, and the clear light of early dawn.

Some say that the experiences of the two sets occur together. Others say they do not. The latter approach is correct. The external signs of smoke and so forth actually precede the experience of the four emptinesses. This is stated in many authoritative tantric scriptures.

The four visions associated with the four "emptinesses" are all experienced as a cloudless sky, with a difference in the color; first white, and then red, black, and finally a clear radiance.

By the time the clear light experience occurs, the three vision-like emptiness experiences [i.e., appearance, proximity and proximate attainment] have already taken place and the vital energies have gathered into the indestructible drop at the heart chakra. The white drop has descended from the crown chakra [during the first emptiness, with the vision of whiteness], the red drop has risen from the navel chakra [during the second emptiness, with the vision of redness], and the two came together at the heart [during the third emptiness, with the vision of darkness].

Although sentient beings other than those possessing the six constituents also experience death and the process of dissolution leading up to the emergence of the clear light, they are not able to recognize or work with the natural dynamic of the situation.

The signs of the dissolution of the elements and the experience of them all take place prior to actual death. One should understand the process well. From the time the first sign occurs one applies whatever methods one is competent in for directing the energies into the central channel. As each of the four signs [indicating the dissolution of the four elements] occurs, one must recognize and confirm the experience, linking mindfulness of the vision of emptiness with the actual occurrence. In the remaining dissolutions one stabilizes the resolution to engage the yogic applications and "blendings."

During the experience of the clear light of death, the subtle energies and consciousness collect into the central channel. The subtle energies enter into the heart chakra, and all coarse activity of the confused mind of duality becomes pacified. A vision like that of a cloudless sky manifests. One must recognize this vision when it occurs, place the mind firmly within it, and apply whatever was achieved through meditation upon the middle view of voidness during one's lifetime.

If during one's lifetime one did not cultivate this ability to place the mind in the view of emptiness, then there will be no way to do so now. Therefore it is fundamental to the success of the bardo yogas that during one's lifetime one cultivates two qualities: the ability to place the mind in a stable understanding of emptiness; and the yogic means of inducing the four blisses. One must apply this technology here for taking "the child clear light" as "the clear light of the path."

Jetsun Milarepa stated,

> The clear light of death is in nature the Dharmakaya; one must recognize it for what it is. To achieve that ability one must have been introduced to it by one's spiritual master. Cultivate knowledge of the essence of the ultimate view, and of the technology for bringing the clear light into the stream of the conventional path.

This fundamental clear light of death is in nature "the mother clear light." One must blend it with "the child clear light of the path."

To gain the ability [to do this at the time of death] one must practice for it in this lifetime. During the waking state one brings the vital energies into the central channel and there causes them to abide and dissolve; one must gain familiarity in this way with the four emptinesses, and particularly "utter emptiness" [i.e., the fourth emptiness, or clear light]. Also, during sleep one blends awareness with the clear light of sleep, no matter how deep one's sleep is. When one trains during the waking and sleeping states in this way, the strength of control over the subtle energies and mind that one achieves will provide one with the power to blend "mother and child clear lights" at the time of death.

If one can recognize the clear light of death in this way and blend with it as instructed, one will be able to recognize the bardo experiences that follow and consequently will be able to apply the yogic technology [for achieving enlightenment in the bardo]. Therefore it is said that the supreme method of implementing the bardo yogas depends upon the ability to recognize and blend with the clear light of death. In fact, there is no "best" way to implement it other than that.

A lesser method is to cultivate the thought, "I am dead. These appearances must be bardo manifestations." However, even though this thought may possibly help one to recognize the fact that one is in the bardo, the realization will be weak.

Likewise one can cultivate meditation on the dissolution of the elements and so forth, as occurs at the time of death [as described earlier]. Then when the four emptinesses of the clear light of death manifest, one can apply whatever samadhi was achieved during one's lifetime. Yet if during one's lifetime one did not learn to direct the vital energies into the central channel, then it is difficult to classify the method [implemented at the time of death] as belonging to the extraordinary category of a highest yoga tantra practice.

Therefore those with interest in these [bardo yogas, which belong to highest yoga tantra practice] should not be like the person who ignores the trunk of the tree and takes only the branches. From the very depths of the marrow of their bones they should aspire to cultivate the yoga of the inner heat and its pure means of bringing the vital energies into the central channel, as was described earlier. During the waking state they should bring the vital energies into the central channel, and cause them to abide and dissolve there. In this way they induce the experience of the four emptinesses. When this practice becomes mature they then learn to retain the clear light of sleep by means of controlling the subtle energies.

After thus cultivating the meditations on the clear light consciousness in the waking state and the clear light consciousness of sleep, one applies the yogic technology for arousing the illusory body. This will empower one with a most wonderful ability to recognize the clear light of death and the ensuing bardo. For all of this, the foundation is the inner heat yoga. Always remember this basic principle.

One recognizes and retains the clear light of death. Then when one begins to pass beyond the clear light and into the bardo, one engages the key points in arousing meditative familiarity and resolution. With these as the guidelines one enters into the bardo with confidence and the positive mind, while engaging the technology for recognizing the bardo visions as illusions, and arising with the illusory body of a tantric mandala deity.

Recognizing the bardo in this way, one determines to achieve a more highly qualified bardo body. The ordinary bardo body by itself is not an adequate vehicle with which to achieve highest spiritual power. The difference comes when one applies a number of factors:

meditating upon oneself as a mandala deity; cultivating meditation on the view of emptiness; cultivating the vision that the world and its inhabitants are like illusory appearances; meditating upon how, just as the dream yoga teaching points to the illusory nature of the dream body, the same principles are applied in the bardo yoga; and so forth. These teachings, drawn from the oral tradition in this way, are termed "the bardo teachings." One engages in them.

It is not certain that the yogic practitioners familiar with these methods will take birth in a womb. They may be born in any of the other three ways. Therefore it is important that one apply the instruction on seeing all appearances as deity manifestations, seeing the body of the deity as an illusion, and seeing the illusory appearances as empty of self-nature.

One cultivates these meditations well. In addition, by cultivating awareness of the parent-like guru as male-female in union, and the mandala deity as male-female in union, etc., a special strength is brought into the application.

Then there is the technique known as "the oath of rebirth." Here one cultivates the aspiration to take rebirth into any of the pure buddha lands.

In the oral tradition teachings of Marpa there is one instruction that speaks of recognizing the bardo, and then sending forth the aspiration to take rebirth in a higher world. This is similar to what we will see later, in the section on consciousness transference.

How to meditate upon the clear light yogas

This is taught under two headings: how one meditates upon the clear light during the waking period; and how to meditate upon the clear light during sleep.

How to meditate upon the clear light during the waking period

The clear light is discussed in two contexts.

The first of these is the general usage. Here it is said that the fundamental reality of being is something free from the extremes of being and non-being. This is the emptiness nature, the "clear light as object." The consciousness that perceives it is the "clear light as subject" [i.e., awareness].

This is the general meaning to the term "clear light." The usage is common to both Hinayana and Mahayana vehicles, to the Paramitayana and Mantrayana vehicles, to all three lower tantra vehicles, and to highest yoga tantra. Thus this is the definition of the clear light in a general sense.

The second usage of the term "clear light" is exclusive to highest yoga tantra. Here there is no difference in the sense of "clear light as object." The difference is in the "clear light as subject," the perceiving mind. Here this is the great innate ecstasy consciousness, which is the specialty of highest yoga tantra. Thus it is called "the exclusive clear light." Its prerequisite is mainly the innate ecstasy consciousness that is aroused by proficiency in the completion stage yogas for bringing the vital energies into the central channel and causing them to abide and dissolve there.

This is not simply the mind of bliss aroused by the melting of the bodhimind substances and placing the mind in non-conceptual meditative absorption free from torpor or agitation, which is a non-conceptual state induced by sublimating some of the vital energies. Even on the generation stage there was some melting produced from the ecstasy of the energy application. This is not what is being used here. One must appreciate these distinctions.

What is being referred to here is the innate ecstasy aroused by means of the inner heat yoga described earlier, known as "the great innate ecstasy of the completion stage." This is conjoined with stabilized awareness of suchness, or emptiness, which gives rise to "the primordial wisdom of ecstasy and emptiness." That is what is here posited as the clear light as "subject." It is the clear light of the path, having the illusory body of the completion stage as its predecessor. Based on prolonged familiarity with that practice, one produces the illusory body, and then uses this in the meditation. This is an exalted dimension of the clear light principle. To engage it one requires the inner basis of the attainment of either the actual illusory body or a proxy. This is then immersed in the clear light.

As for the stages of merging into the clear light, most of the oral tradition teachings [on the Six Yogas] are somewhat unclear on this point. Some of them, however, do provide excellent documentation.

These latter recommend that one visualize oneself as the maṇḍala deity, male and female in sexual union, the "wheel of truth" chakra at the heart, the central channel running through it. One meditates on a blue mantric syllable HUM standing on a sun disk located there. Lights emanate from this and purify the inanimate universe. The universe melts into clear light, which absorbs into the animate universe. These then melt into clear light and into oneself as the mandala deity. The female aspect melts into the male of the mandala deity.

Then from one's crown downward and feet upward one melts into light, which is absorbed into the syllable HUM at one's heart.

The syllable HUM then melts into light from the bottom upward, beginning with the U vowel underneath melting into the AH, that into the HA, that into its own head, that into the crescent moon above, that into the drop, and that into the nada above it. In this way all is absorbed into the center of the central channel at the heart chakra.

One places the mind firmly there, causing the energies from the side channels of rasana and lalana to enter, abide and dissolve within the central channel, arousing the four emptinesses, and giving rise to the amazing clear light consciousness of the path. When this occurs one observes the mind of the great innate ecstasy and then holds to it.

As said earlier, this process for both the illusory body and clear light yogas is wonderfully elucidated in the oral tradition of the Arya Cycle of Guhyasamaja teachings. The manner of merging with the clear light as described immediately above is also similar to the special dhyana for entering into the clear light as taught in the Guhyasamaja tradition of The Five Stages. Therefore my presentation above is somewhat adorned by the mode of explanation found in the oral tradition of the Guhyasamaja system.

Previously in the meditations on the inner heat one absorbed the vital energies into the central channel and gave rise to the innate ecstasy. Here again one directs the energies into the central channel and invokes the stages of dissolution as explained in that earlier process, giving rise to the innate great ecstasy and eventually the clear light.

If one is unable to do this, then whatever familiarity with the dissolution process one has achieved should here be applied.

I have written on this technology in greater depth elsewhere.

How to meditate upon the clear light during sleep

If the situation is such that one can retain the clear light of sleep by means of controlling the vital energies, then as explained before one does this and engages in the dream yogas. Retaining the clear light of sleep is the supreme method for working in the dream state. To accomplish the application in this way is in accord with how most previous lineage masters have taught on the subject.

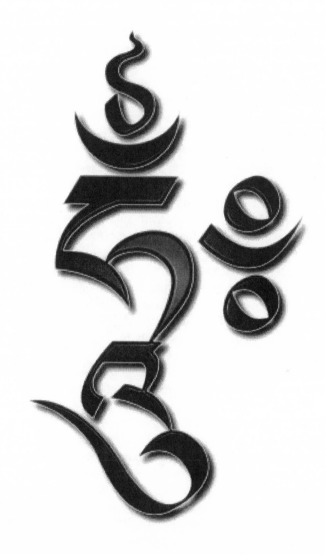

The syllable HUM

Before engaging in the practice one should follow a healthy diet, dress warmly, and so forth. There is also a tradition of cutting one's sleep for two or three days, but this is not always done. The important thing is to make one's sleep more light. When sleep is heavy it is more difficult for the novice in the practice to retain the clear light of sleep. When sleep is subtle, this clear light is more easily retained. One wants to create the latter condition. Then when the practice becomes mature one may succeed under the former condition. At that time one will not have to cut one's sleep [to create a lighter sleep state], although one may do so in order to observe the progress of the yoga in conditions of deep sleep.

The practice here is to engage in devotional exercises focusing upon the Three Jewels of Refuge during the day and evening, and make *torma* offerings to the Dharma Protectors. Send forth prayers that one may recognize the clear light of sleep, and that obstructions to this may be mitigated. One meditates on oneself as the mandala deity. Also, one meditates on guru yoga and sends forth many prayers for blessing power to assist in the effort to retain the clear light of sleep.

Then one makes firm the resolution that as one goes to sleep one will recognize and retain the four emptinesses that occur prior to the emergence of dreams. One lies on one's right side in the sleeping lion posture, with one's head to the north, back to the east, face to the west and feet to the south, one's right foot on top of the left, and right arm tucked underneath the body. One visualizes oneself as the mandala deity, and envisions a blue four-petalled lotus at one's heart chakra, the central channel running through it, a blue mantric syllable *HUM* at its center.

Here there are the two traditions: that of placing the mantric syllables *AH, NU, TA* and *RA* respectively on the four lotus petals, with *HUM* at the center; and that of using only the syllable *HUM*.

In the former case, the *AH* is placed in the east, *NU* in the south, *TA* in the west and *RA* in the north. One first places the awareness on *AH*; then when sleep is about to begin one switches awareness to *NU*, and there occurs the first "emptiness," known simply as "empty" and as "appearance." One places awareness on *TA*, and the second "emptiness," known as "very empty" and as "proximity," occurs. One places awareness on *RA*; the experience of "great empty" and "proximate attainment" occurs. Finally one places awareness at the syllable *HUM* at the center of the central channel; the fourth emptiness, known as "utterly empty," arises.

It is said that one should meditate on these mantric syllables in conjunction with the occurrence of the four emptinesses in this way. However, although some teachers give this instruction, it seems to me that they are overlooking the principle that envisioning the syllables at the center of the central channel is what causes the vital energies to be drawn into the heart chakra, giving rise to the experiences of entering, abiding and dissolving, which in turn induces experience of the four emptinesses. Therefore although it is said that the mantric syllables are to be envisioned at the heart chakra, it is not stated sufficiently clearly that these must be inside the central channel of *avadhuti* at the center of the heart chakra. Hence even though there is mention made [in those oral traditions] of linking these auxiliary mantric syllables to the process of the "emptinesses," in fact the manner in which most lineages today present them undermines the basis of accomplishing the desired result. Therefore there is no significant advantage in using the syllables *AH NU TA RA*, and it is acceptable to dispense with them altogether [i.e., to simply visualize the syllable *HUM* at the center, as described above]. The important point, in either of the two methods, is that the mind is placed at the center of the central channel inside the heart chakra.

The yogis who engage in this practice of retaining the clear light of sleep are of two types: those who have previously achieved samadhi able to abide in firm meditation, and those who have not.

In the latter case, on going to sleep the yogi cultivates the instructions as above and attempts to rest in that samadhi once sleep sets in. However, this will only last a short time. He must arouse the awareness that he is in the sleep state [in order to pursue the concentration], but this is difficult under these conditions. Thus he will be unable to remain in the contemplation for very long.

If one goes to sleep without first bringing the vital energies under control then one will not be able to cut off the subtle passage of breath through the two nostrils, and as a result one will not arouse an actual experience of even a semblance of the fourth emptiness. The qualified experience will not arise, and thus the actuality of retaining the clear light of sleep will not be achieved.

The practitioners who have achieved the *samadhi* of firm placement are also of two types. The first of these have, during the waking state, cultivated a thorough familiarity with the process of the inner heat yogas. By means of it they have brought the vital energies into *dhuti*, causing them to enter, abide and dissolve there, and given rise to the experience of the [four] emptinesses. In this case while going to sleep they cultivate the visualizations as explained above, with the syllable *HUM* at the center of *dhuti* inside the heart chakra. Within two or three days they are able to recognize the stages of dissolution into the four emptinesses of sleep, and will gain the ability to retain the clear light of sleep.

Even if one is not able to induce the experiences of the four emptinesses during the waking state, one should in general make firm the samadhi characterized as blissful, radiant and beyond conceptuality. One then engages the above visualization at the time of going to bed and attempts to recognize the dissolutions. If still these [four emptinesses] are not recognized, one continues to cultivate samadhi during the daytime, and eventually this will carry over into the sleep state. Here stable samadhi conjoined with ecstasy is enough; there is no need to bring the vital energies into the central channel.

However, in such a situation the practice could not be said to be a highest yoga tantra method for inducing retention of the clear light of sleep. The degree to which one can hold the visualization inside the heart chakra is the degree to which the seeds of success in the practice are planted.

The power to experience samadhi in sleep by means of cultivating ordinary samadhi powers [during the waking state], even when conjoined with meditation on the view of suchness, will induce only a conventional experience of the clear light of sleep [i.e., the experience will only be on the coarse level of consciousness]. It will not induce the experience of the clear light of sleep as described in highest yoga tantra [i.e., on the most subtle level of consciousness]. Hence it will not qualify as a practice of highest yoga tantra. Nonetheless, meditating in that way and envisioning the mantric syllable (or syllables) and so forth as explained above does plant the instincts for unfoldment in that direction.

This "shared" samadhi [i.e., common to highest tantra and other paths] can produce the ability to dwell in actual samadhi during the sleep state, and can be conjoined with awareness of the view of emptiness in order to give rise to an experience of the "clear light of the shared path." However, it is not the clear light consciousness induced through practice of highest yoga tantra.

As explained earlier, one should meditate on the heart chakra in order to establish energy control, which in turn gives rise to the experience of the four emptinesses [of entering into the sleep state].

In general it is said that the drop which supports the experience of the deep sleep state naturally resides in the heart chakra. When one utilizes this as a path one can induce an amazing experience of the clear light of sleep. Even when it is not utilized as a path, the vital energies naturally withdraw into this drop when one goes to sleep. Hence if during the waking state one cultivates the ability to bring the vital energies into the central channel, and when going to sleep applies the meditations described above, maintaining the visualizations inside the central channel at the heart chakra, it becomes quite easy to bring the energies into the central channel at the heart chakra by means of the techniques explained earlier.

The stages in which this occurs begin with the experience of a vision like that of a mirage of shimmering water. This dissolves, and then a vision like that of all-pervading smoke arises. That subsides, and there is an appearance of many small flickering lights, like fireflies in the air. That subsides, and there is an appearance of a steadily glowing light, like that of a butterlamp undisturbed by the movement of wind.

That subsides, and the white drop descends. There is an appearance of whiteness, like moonlight in a clear night sky. This is the experience of "appearance," and the first "emptiness." Then there is the appearance of red or reddish yellow, like sunlight in a clear sky, pervading everything. This is the emergence of the experience of "proximity" and the second emptiness. Next there is a vision of utter darkness, like that of a pitch black sky; this is the third emptiness, and the state of "proximate attainment." Prior to this one had retained consciousness, but here one swoons into darkness, and all awareness and memory fade away. However, this is not a fault; for the more strongly one loses consciousness, the better becomes the opportunity for practice. The more intense one's vision of darkness, the more dominant will be the clear light consciousness when it emerges. Such is the state known as "the great emptiness" and "proximate attainment."

Finally this experience of "proximate attainment" subsides, and one revives from the depths of unconsciousness. There is a sense of clear light, like that of the sky at dawn, when there is neither sun,

moon nor darkness. This is the experience known as "utter emptiness" and as "clear light." One places one's awareness within it and
retains it for as long as possible. Here one engages in the methods of
avoiding either slipping into the dream state or waking up [while
cultivating the clear light of sleep].

I have written on these techniques separately in my commentary
to the Marpa tradition of Guhyasamaja.

These "four emptinesses" are linked to the four blisses. The fourth
emptiness here is the experience of the clear light of sleep, and is concomitant with the experience of the innate supreme ecstasy.

Here there is this bliss, and also that induced by means of placing
the mind in the state of beyond conceptuality. Although the name
"bliss" is applied equally to both, a differentiation should be made.
The former is like seeing the sky itself, whereas the latter is like seeing a mere similitude.

This great ecstasy arises, and one simultaneously focuses without
mental wandering on mindfulness of the view of suchness, as explained earlier. This is the state of consciousness so lavishly praised
in highest yoga tantra as "inseparable ecstasy and void." This state of
being is subtle, and lesser absorptions are easily mistaken for it. Therefore it is important to observe the experience carefully.

Some oral tradition teaching lineages here omit the work with the
first three emptinesses. Others speak of the four emptinesses, but have
no clear explanation of how they are to be recognized and retained.

In some oral traditions coming from Lama Ngokpa no clear method
of recognizing these experiences is given. However, [Ngokpa recommends that] these can be learned from *A Compendium of Tantric Experiences* (Skt. *Charya melapaka pradipa*).[53] Here that text states,

> The aggregates dissolve into the subtle elements. The subtle ele-
> ments dissolve into consciousness. Consciousness in turn dissolves
> into mind. Mind dissolves into unknowing.
>   Having experienced these states, one enters into sleep. At that
> time, consciousness and mind dissolve into unknowing, and all
> memory and awareness are temporarily lost. After that the state
> of unknowingness fades, and the clear light, in nature primordial
> wisdom, emerges. When that [i.e., the clear light] is released, the
> energies move spontaneously by their natural inclination, giving
> rise to dreams. For as long as the mind does not waver, retain it in
> the sleep state, and place it in observance of the clear light of sleep.

The authoritative writings of the mahasiddhas, in explaining the
four emptinesses of entering into the sleep state, advocate this

approach of recognizing and working with the clear light of sleep. There is no more authoritative scriptural source for the practice. Thus one should understand it in this way.

In the above passage the words "the aggregates dissolve..." refer to the appearance of the coarse aspects of the aggregates.

The "subtle elements dissolve..." refers to everything dissolving into the energies. Here, earth energies dissolve into those of water, water into fire, and fire into air. Then this dissolves into the consciousness known as "the first appearance," which is what is meant by the words "dissolve into consciousness" [in the above passage]. This [dissolution into consciousness] refers to the first emptiness.

Also, here the word "mind" refers to the appearance of the vision known as "proximity." "Dissolves" refers to the moment when that consciousness [i.e., "appearance"] withdraws into the mind of "proximity." "Unknowing" refers to the experience of "proximate attainment." "Having experienced these states..." has the sense of consciously mixing or blending with these three "emptinesses" as they arise at the time of entering into sleep.

The process of recognizing these states is taught in *A Compendium of Wisdom Diamonds* (Skt. *Vajrajnana samucchaya*)and is explained in *A Compendium of Tantric Experiences*. My comments follow their direction.

The words "at that time..." refer to the time of sleep. The words "consciousness and mind dissolve into unknowing..." refer to one successively melting into the next. "After that..." refers to the occasion following that of "proximate attainment." The words "the state of unknowingness fades..." is in reference to awakening from the darkness of unconsciousness and is characterized by the experience of a light like that of dawn with a clear sky. No other signs occur after this.

Here in the translation by Chak Lotsawa we see the words of the above passage rendered somewhat differently: "The energies move spontaneously by their natural inclination; for as long as no dreams occur...." This is a good way of expressing the idea. The meaning is that after the samadhi of the clear light of sleep is released, the mind slips out of the clear light experience. The energies then begin to stir of their own inclination, and one enters into the dream state. The passage, "For as long as the mind does not waver..." means that until dreams naturally begin to arise one should remain in the clear light absorption.

However, if the clear light of sleep cannot be retained by means of energy control, then one can generate samadhi at the time of going to sleep and try to focus it on the clear light. One should keep in mind that the samadhi must recognize the processes of the first three "emptinesses," or else the clear light will not be recognized. Otherwise, the clear light experienced in that samadhi will not be the clear light of sleep, even if the samadhi is vibrantly radiant. Moreover, as a prelude to the first "emptiness," one should have been aware of the visions of the mirage, smoke, and so forth, that indicate the withdrawal of the elemental energies. If these are not recognized, no real clarity or focus can be established during the application.

In training to work with the clear light of sleep it helps to understand the clear lights of experience and realization; and the two clear lights characterized as "thin" and "thick."

As for invoking the power of a vibrantly radiant non-conceptual samadhi when dreams occur, this relies on retaining the clear light of sleep. However, even if one had learned many instructions on the methods of retaining the clear light of sleep, these will be of no avail if one utilizes a samadhi of sleep that does not follow the process [of dissolutions and the experiences of the emptinesses]. The mind will not be sufficiently stable to retain the application. Therefore the instructions on how to train during both waking and sleep states must be correctly understood. For this the principles of the practice as outlined in the excellent writings of the Aryas, master and disciple [i.e., Nagarjuna and Aryadeva], are most valuable, and in one's practice one should hold to them closely, regarding them as deeply cherished oral instructions.

If one engages the above methodology for retaining the clear light of sleep but the movement of vital energies renders the effort unsuccessful, then one should engage in the manner of working within dreams as taught in wonderful detail in the Marpa lineage of the Guhyasamaja oral instruction teachings.

The branches of that path, which include the practices of consciousness transference and forceful projection

This section of the tradition explains two techniques, namely, those for consciousness transference, and those for forceful entry to a new residence.

Consciousness transference

This instruction on the methods for transferring consciousness to a higher realm is a unique feature of highest yoga tantra. It is taught in the *Sambhuta Tantra*, which is an explanatory tantra shared by both the Chakrasamvara and Hevajra systems. It is also taught in *The Diamond Sky Dancer Tantra* (Skt. *Vajradaka tantra*), which is an explanatory tantra associated exclusively with Chakrasamvara. Further, we see it referred to in various root tantras, including both *The Root Tantra of Chakrasamvara* (Skt. *Shri chakrasamvara mula tantra*) and *The Arising of Samvara Tantra* (Skt. *Samvarodaya tantra*), as well as *The Four Seats Tantra* (Skt. *Shri chaturpitha tantra*). We also see it referred to in *The Book of Manjushri's Direct Instructions* and other such works. Those who wish to understand it fully would do well to read these authoritative sources and their commentaries.

The beneficial effects of this path are elucidated in *The Diamond Sky Dancer Tantra*:

> Killing a brahmin every day,
> Committing any of the five inexpiable acts,
> Stealing and even rape:
> All these karmas are purified through this path.
> One sheds the clothing of guilt for evil deeds done
> And goes far beyond the faults of the world.

Although translated [into Tibetan] slightly differently, this same passage is also found in both *The Mystic Kiss Tantra* (Skt. *Chaturyogini samputa tantra*) and *The Four Seats Tantra*. As it is such a quintessential precept, one should apply oneself to it well.

It is said that this path both purifies and liberates. It liberates from rebirth into any of the three lower realms; and it purifies the mind of negative karmic seeds that ripen as lower rebirths. This is the explanation given in *A Harvest of Oral Tradition Teachings*.

As for the time at which the actual consciousness transference should be made, this is described as follows in *The Diamond Sky Dancer Tantra*:

> Perform transference when the time comes;
> To do so earlier is to kill a deity.
> As a result of killing a deity,
> One will certainly burn in hell.
> Therefore the wise make effort
> To know the signs of death.

This same thing is said in both *The Four Seats Tantra* and *The Mystic Kiss Tantra*. To transfer the consciousness out of the body prematurely is equivalent to suicide; and as one is cultivating the yoga of envisioning oneself as a mandala deity, it is equivalent to killing a tantric deity. Moreover, if one holds the mantra precepts, then suicide is prohibited by the eighth root precept. One should know that to transgress it will result in rebirth in the hells. Therefore it is important to understand the correct time for the application.

To know this well, one should make the effort to learn the path of reading the signs of death. When one sees the appearance of the signs of death, and also sees signs indicating that the methods for turning death away will not work, this is the time for the application of the actual consciousness transference.

The text *A Commentary to the Four Seats Tantra* (Skt. *Shri chaturpitha tika*) by Bhavabhadra states that one should train in the method at least six months before one's death. Therefore it is important to become skilled in reading the signs indicating the unfolding of one's lifespan.

Moreover, *The Four Seats Tantra* states,

> The best time to train in the transference yogas
> Is before one becomes afflicted with illness.

As said here, it is best to undertake the training when one is not weakened by disease. Otherwise, once a debilitating disease has set in, it becomes difficult to effect the transfer of consciousness as desired, even if one previously had made some progress in the training.

If one thinks to apply consciousness transference simply [as a means of ending one's life] because of terrible sufferings due to age, or unbearable pain due to an illness, this also is said to be inappropriate. Even though some traditions do condone the former situation, it is a great mistake.

The actual teaching on the yoga of consciousness transference involves two main trainings.

The first of these is described in *The Diamond Sky Dancer Tantra* as follows:

> One purifies the limit of the residence.
> Having purified it, one implements the transference.
> Otherwise, there will be no benefit.

Here "the limit of the residence" refers to the human body, which is the "residence" within which pleasure and pain are experienced. To try and engage the transference yogas without first having purified the body by means of the inner heat doctrine explained earlier will produce no meaningful results. This was stated by Bhavabhadra in his commentary. Thus meditation on the inner heat yoga can here be regarded as a condition for success in the transference yoga. *The Diamond Sky Dancer Tantra* states,

> One ties the doors with the vase breathing technique
> And purifies the channel which is a door.

The *Four Seats Tantra* and also the *Sambhuta Tantra* say much the same thing. The meaning is that one meditates on the vase breathing technique, and by means of it withdraws the vital energies flowing to the various doors, such as those of the sensory powers, redirecting these energies into the central channel.

Previously the practitioners of vase breathing were described as being of three types: best, medium, and least qualified. It is sometimes said that even the third of these [the least qualified] can successfully implement the transference yogas. This indicates a misunderstanding of the tantric treatises.

Here one blocks the exit of consciousness by any gate other than the golden aperture at the crown. The other eight gates are blocked, and consciousness is directed to leave the body via the golden gate at the crown.

To accomplish transference in such a way as to acquire the supreme basis of a knowledge holder of tantric activities, one requires the instructions as provided in the tantric scriptures [mentioned earlier]. What is required is a qualified meditational application, as described in the tantric literature, for directing the movement of consciousness out of the body.

There are a number of oral tradition teachings on the subject. That known as "consciousness transference by means of the four techniques" and also the Ngok lineage (Tib. *rNgog lugs*) of consciousness transference provide wonderfully detailed presentations of the meditations involved. However, in this tradition [i.e., the Six Yogas of Naropa], the oral transmissions of most lamas present the instructions of consciousness transference based on oral transmission alone. I will speak in brief on what is said by them.

What is the best mandala deity upon which to meditate in conjunction with the consciousness transference yogas? Most gurus recommend that this be whatever is the principal mandala deity one has cultivated in meditation. Alternatively, *The Mystic Kiss Tantra* and *The Four Seats Tantra* each recommend a specific deity practice for the techniques that they present, and one can utilize these. But to write on these other systems here would require too many words, and therefore I will not do so.

Here the oral tradition suggests that one should visualize oneself as one's mandala deity, and bring the vital energies into a kiss at either the secret place chakra or the navel chakra. One then envisions the red *AH*-stroke syllable at the navel chakra; at the heart chakra, a dark blue *HUM*; and at the crown aperture, a white *KSHA*.[54]

Now one pulls up forcefully on the vital energies from below. These strike the *AH*-stroke syllable at the navel chakra, which then rises and strikes the *HUM* at the heart. This rises and strikes the *KSHA* at the crown. Then the process is reversed: the *HUM* comes back down to the heart chakra; and the *AH* comes back down to the navel chakra.

Here sometimes it is said that the *AH*-stroke syllable dissolves into *HUM* [and that into the *KSHA*] during the upward movement. The approach as described above is more effective.

One should apply oneself to this training until the signs of accomplishment manifest, such as a small blister appearing on the crown of the head, a sensation of itching, and so forth.

As for the actual application [i.e., at the time of death], here some lamas recommend that one place the body in the *tsig-bu* position, with the two arms wrapped around the knees. As preliminaries one takes Refuge, generates the bodhimind, and then meditates upon oneself as being the mandala deity. In the space in front of one's crown, an armspan or half an armspan in distance, one visualizes one's root guru, in aspect inseparable from [i.e., appearing in the form of] one's meditational deity. One offers reverent prayers to him or her.

Now one turns one's concentration to the three mantric syllables: the red *AH*-stroke at the navel chakra; blue *HUM* at the heart chakra; and white *KSHA* at the crown. The energies are forcefully drawn up from below, causing the *AH*-stroke syllable to rise up the central channel from the navel chakra and melt into the *HUM* at the heart chakra. One recites the mantra *AH HIK* several times. The *HUM* syllable moves up. One recites the mantra *AH HIK* twenty times, and it continues up to the throat chakra.

One turns the attention to the syllable *KSHA* at the mouth of the Brahma aperture, silhouetted against a background of pure white sky-like light, like an object in a roof window. One recites *AH HIK*

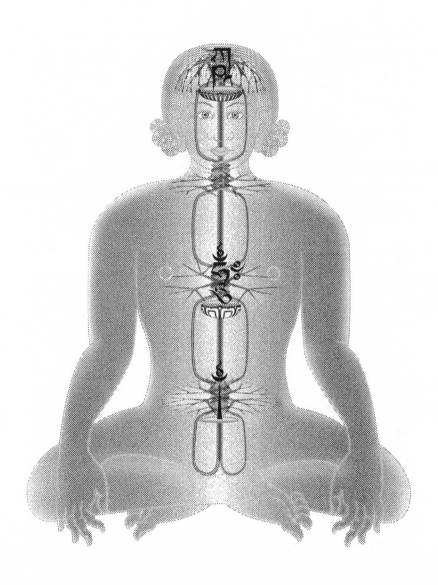

Channels, chakras and mantric syllables
for the yoga of consciousness transference

forcefully five times, and the syllable HUM shoots out the Brahma aperture and melts into the heart of the guru inseparable from one's mandala deity. Rest awareness there in the state beyond conceptuality.

Such is the process as taught by the gurus of the lineage. It accords with the brief outline of the consciousness transference doctrine given in *The Four Seats Tantra*. That tantra and its commentary are authoritative sourceworks. As they point out, one's understanding of the technique of consciousness transference is benefited by understanding the details of the practice, such as the seats of the two principal syllables mentioned, the exact site where the two syllables are placed, the manner of placing the syllables upright and in reverse,[55] the application of energy control and recitation at the two occasions of upward transference, and the special techniques of yogic application. If one can understand the process well and apply oneself to the training, the desired effects will be produced.

Then there is also the oral tradition teaching for transferring consciousness to rebirth in a paradise, and the technique for transferring consciousness to a rebirth that can act as the basis of a supreme master of tantric activities. For this one must be able to apply the force of an exclusive samadhi in order to prevent consciousness from leaving the body by any of the other eight gates, and direct it to transfer via the golden gate. If one is able to control the vital energies upon which the subtle consciousness rides, and thus prevent them from flowing to the other eight gates, then one will be able to prevent the consciousness that rides upon the energies from transferring by any of the undesirable eight.[56]

For this one should know the key points in meditating upon mantric syllables in order to close the gates, and also how to use the vase breathing technique in order to withdraw the vital energies from the sensory gates. These are key points. Unfortunately it is rare to find a manual on the process that provides real clarity on these issues.

Numerous masters of the past have recommended that the [eight gates] be closed with the red AH-stroke mantric syllable, like that at the navel chakra. This accords with the passage in the *Sambhuta Tantra* wherein it is said, "That seed syllable is the red one." The same instruction is given in the scripture *A Harvest of Oral Tradition Teachings*, which comments that only the red AH-stroke syllable is to be used.

We do see other approaches, such as, for example, using a red syllable HUM. Some teachers comment that this is based on the *Four Seats Tantra*, which speaks of placing a syllable at each of the nine gates. The syllable mentioned is a red *HUM*. However, this interpretation is a misunderstanding of that tantric scriptural passage.

Forceful projection to a new residence

The sensory powers of the eye and so forth are likened to a house, and the entire body-base supporting the senses is likened to a town. Therefore the word "residence" is used.

As the Prajnaparamita literature puts it, the expression "projection into another residence" is used because one projects consciousness into the undeteriorated corpse of another person; like entering into a foreign village, one projects one's consciousness into that residence. The instruction for this process is a specialty of highest yoga tantra and is taught extensively in many female tantras, and also is mentioned in every male tantra.

What is the nature of the vessels who are able to project consciousness in this way? What is the purpose of the practice? And what is the manner of effecting the projection?

The vessels who are able to accomplish forceful projection

For both consciousness transference and forceful projection, the person doing the practice should have received the initiations and maintained the tantric precepts and commitments. The reasons are much the same as with [why these conditions should be present for training in] the generation stage yogas.

With all three practices—consciousness transference, forceful projection [into a corpse], and projecting someone out of their body into one's own body—one requires the ability to block the flow of energies by placing mantric syllables at the gates, and also the ability to purify the gates by means of using the vase breathing technique to direct the vital energies into the central channel. And one needs the ability to control the red element, the *AH*-stroke syllable at the navel chakra, by means of the inner heat yogas and to utilize it to arouse the consciousness that rides upon the subtle energies, represented by the *HUM* at the heart chakra.

This appears to be the intent expressed in original and commentarial tantric literature, including the *Diamond Sky Dancer Tantra*, the *Four Seats Tantra*, and the commentaries to them by Bhavabhadra, as well as the *Mystic Kiss Tantra* and its commentary, *A Harvest of Oral Tradition Teachings*. The ability to project one's own or another's consciousness requires the presence of those factors mentioned above. It also requires a particular training in energy control and the transformative nature of the energies thus effected.

To learn more on this subject, one can refer to other sources.

The purpose of the practice

The reasons for performing forceful projection into another residence can be multifold. For example, there are those of inauspicious lineage who find that they are unable to accomplish great deeds for the benefit of the world due to physical limitations, and thus may feel it expedient to acquire a more appropriate body. Also, perhaps a physical illness renders one unable to benefit oneself or others, and therefore one is moved to acquire a healthy body. Similarly, one may be afflicted by old age and thus be moved to acquire a youthful body.

For these and similar reasons the technique of "forceful projection into another residence" is utilized.

The manner of effecting the projection

The lineage gurus have outlined three modes of applying the yoga of forceful projection.

In the first of these the practitioner must have acquired control over the subtle levels of energy and consciousness. He must have a vision of greatly benefiting others in this lifetime, and be moved by immeasurable compassion for all living beings. On that basis he implements the yoga of forceful projection into another residence.

With an attendant he takes up the practice in a solitary place, avoids all distracting activities, prepares an altar to the mandala deities, arranges offerings, and sets the limits of the retreat place.

In front of his meditation seat he constructs a mandala on a black base, and stands a human skull-cup at its center, the syllable *HUM* clearly written in it with chalk.

Within the sphere of envisioning himself as the mandala deity, he offers the seven-limbed devotion and then turns his meditation to the mantric syllable *HUM* at his heart. When the breath passes exclusively through the right nostril he imagines the syllable *HUM* at the heart being projected out with the flowing airs. This leaves by the right nostril and melts into the *HUM* in the skull cup. One does not inhale the airs again, but retains the exhalation. When one can no longer retain the exhalation, one slowly inhales the airs again. The process of exhalation is then repeated.

After persisting in this method for some time, signs of progress will begin to manifest. For example, the skull cup will shake, move or jump around on the mandala table of its own accord.

To practice the technique one first acquires a fresh, undisintegrated human corpse of a person who did not die from serious wounds or a debilitating illness. Alternatively, the body of certain animals can be used for the training.

One washes the corpse with fresh water, adorns it with beautiful ornaments, and places it in the crossed-legged posture on the mandala platform that was constructed earlier. One visualizes the mantric syllable *HUM*, the support of consciousness, at both one's own heart and that of the corpse. One breathes out the syllable *HUM* at one's heart; it exits via the right nostril, and enters the body of the corpse via the left nostril, melting into the *HUM* at its heart. One repeats this process over and over, until eventually the corpse begins to breathe and become animated. These are signs that the ability to effect the practice has been acquired, and one is at the threshold of the real practice.

When one is ready for the actual application, one releases the retreat limits that had been set and searches for a human corpse having the prerequisite signs. As before, one places it on the mandala platform, the face pointing toward oneself. It is decorated with ornaments and so forth. One then generates the vision of oneself as the mandala deity, leaves behind all thoughts of attachment to the ordinary physical body, generates the vision of the illusory nature of all phenomena that appear in the world, and transcends all instincts of conceiving the world as ordinary. Within this sphere one makes the sacrificial *torma* offering (Tib. *gtor ma*) to the gurus and the Dharma Protectors, and sends out supplications that hindrances may not arise.

Now one visualizes oneself and the corpse as being tantric deities, a mantric syllable *HUM* at the heart of each. One faces the corpse squarely and breathes out, with the airs passing through the right nostril. The *HUM* at one's heart exits one's body via the right nostril and enters into the body of the corpse via its left nostril. The forces of subtle energies and mind are brought into play in the process of moving the syllable *HUM*, and the airs are expelled forcefully. Eventually the corpse will be resuscitated and will begin to breathe.

When this happens, one has a beautiful friend offer it appropriate food and tend to it.[57] For half a month it is kept hidden inside; and until this new "residence" becomes steady, one also keeps one's old body hidden inside the hut. Then one can cremate the old body in a tantric fire ritual, have the ashes mixed with clay and pressed into holy images, and so forth, in order to show respect to it for the kind service that it had rendered to one. One then takes up one's new life in the newly acquired body, and performs great deeds for the benefit of living beings.

This is the method of "forceful projection into another residence" as taught by the lineage gurus. Different [Indian] tantric scriptures and treatises teach similar methods, without the need for all the details found in the oral tradition described above.

A question of ethics becomes relevant in the application of these doctrines, similar to that which arose in the doctrine of consciousness transference, wherein it was said that to project consciousness out of one's body prematurely is equal to killing a deity or human. Here, however, heavy language of this nature is not used. There is no question of killing or suicide, for [unlike in consciousness transference, here] one does not actually die. It is not like causing oneself to die prematurely, as in an early application of consciousness transference, and thus the parallel cannot be drawn. Here the "death" that is experienced by the yogi or yogini is not a complete death with all the features of a conventional passing. And even though there is forceful projection into another "residence," there is no rebirth in the conventional sense of being born from one of the four types of birth, such as from the womb, from an egg, and so forth. Thus there is no fully characterized rebirth. Furthermore, although the period between the time that consciousness is projected out of one's body until it has entered into the new body may be termed an in-between state [and thus a bardo], it is not a fully characterized bardo of becoming. Moreover, in ordinary death and rebirth there is a total loss of memory of the past life; here there is none of this memory loss.

If one wishes to understand the principles of this extraordinary practice more fully, they are to be found in the teachings of the Guhyasamaja oral transmission teaching known as the "Oral Tradition of the Body-Form of Glorious Guhyasamaja" (Tib. *dPal 'dus pa'i sku lus kyi man ngag*).

Although there are said to be traditions of both forcefully projecting one's own consciousness into another residence [as described above], and forcefully projecting the consciousness of someone else into one's own body [in order to offer it to them], this second tradition is not publicly taught by the gurus. Therefore I will not write of it here.

The methods and activities for enhancing the path

To accomplish enlightenment in this lifetime one must engage in the special tantric activities for enhancing the path. Here there are those tantric activities associated with the generation stage yogas, and those associated with the completion stage yogas. *The Clear Lamp* (Skt. *Pradipoddyotana*) speaks of the activities on both of these stages as being of three types, simply called "with embellishment," "without embellishment," and "utterly without embellishment."[58]

The tone of the term "tantric activities" here is that one enters the door of thoroughly understanding the self-nature principle, and through it utilizes the objects of sensuality in general, and a wisdom consort in particular. In this way there arises a wondrous realization of suchness.

Hence "activity utterly without embellishment" refers to the wisdom consort, the jnanamudra that is the seal of wisdom, the knowledge lady.

As for the other two of the three ["with embellishment" and "without embellishment"], they involve the sensual karmamudra, or activities utilizing an actual sexual partner.

The manner of implementing these is also of three types: the expanded practice, which includes singing, dancing, and so forth; the medium version, in which these are abbreviated; and the third mode, in which one dispenses with all external embellishments.[59]

The time for these tantric activities is also threefold: when one is attempting to manifest the illusory body for the first time; when the illusory body has been achieved and one is attempting to train in the clear light yogas; and when the great union state of a trainee has been attained and one is attempting to master the yogas of the great union beyond training.

These methods are taught because during these phases in the training one requires an oral tradition teaching containing the complete details of the practice. I have mentioned them in brief merely in order to lay instincts for the practice [on the mindstreams of the readers]. To address these issues here would require too many words. Those who want to know more on the subject should search the oral tradition teachings on the Guhyasamaja Tantra.

The manner of actualizing the results

After the stage of the great union of a trainee has been achieved one enters into meditation on the clear light, through which all instincts of the confused state of grasping at duality are washed away. Then at the time of finally manifesting the Dharmakaya, the illusory body of the practitioner on the stage of the great union of a trainee utterly transforms and becomes an illusory body of the great union beyond training. That illusory body will not falter for as long as samsara exists.

At that point the clear light as an object possessing the two pure qualities becomes the Uncompounded Dharmakaya. The clear light as subject [i.e., as the perceiving mind] becomes what is known as the Jnana Dharmakaya, or Wisdom Truth Body, and as the Mahasukhakaya, or "Great Ecstasy Body."

The support of that [Dharmakaya state] is the Rupakaya, created solely from [the most subtle levels of] energy and mind of the form-aspect of the being. This is the Sambhogakaya.

These two "bodies"—the Dharmakaya [Truth Body] and Rupakaya [Form Body]—both have the same essential natures, but dramatically distinct existential presences. Therefore sometimes we see the Rupakaya also referred to as the "Body of Non-dual Wisdom."

[The last expression above has given rise to some misinterpretations. For example,] we see it said that the Rupakaya is not collected by the stream of being of the person accomplishing buddhahood, but rather is collected by the stream of being of those to be trained. Others speak of the Rupakaya being other than mind, and formed from physical matter. Then there is the saying that at the time of resultant buddhahood there is no primordial wisdom. None of this is especially useful.

Here this illusory body of the stage of the great union transforms into the Nirmanakaya, and is able to send forth countless emanations.

Epilogue

[Of the two fundamental texts that serve as the basis of the Six Yogas of Naropa,] here there is *The Early Compendium Root Text* (Tib. *Ka dpe rtsa ba'i sdom snga ma*), and *The Later Compendium Root Text* (Tib. *Ka dpe rtsa ba'i sdom phyi ma*). It seems that there are two internal contradictions with the former text. Some traditions purport that the second one was compiled by Lama Marpa himself. There is also a commentary to the oral instruction tradition of the Guhyasamaja Tantra that is attributed to Lama Marpa. We see such statements made, but it is difficult to ascertain their veracity.

Another work attributed to Lama Marpa is entitled *Eight Instructions in Verse and Prose* (Tib. *Tshig rkang brgyad ma*), which blends verse and prose in its presentation. Then there is *The Vajra Song of the Six Dharmas* (Tib. *Chos drug rdo rje'i mgur*). However, these two are only intended to plant the seeds of the oral tradition teachings, and are too terse to do much more than that.

There are also several oral traditions of the six yogas of Naropa based on revealed "treasure texts" that have appeared. These do not inspire much confidence.[60]

Marpa transmitted his lineage [of the Six Yogas of Naropa] to three of his disciples: Ngokton, Tsurton, and Milarepa. In turn, Milarepa transmitted his lineages to two main disciples: Chojey Gampopa and Rechungpa. The lineage descending from Gampopa multiplied into many different forms, each with its own specialty, uniqueness and individual views on the different practices. I gathered the essence of all of these through personal effort and experience.

The instruction on the inner heat yoga comes to us through Tilopa, who commented that this was the transmission of the mahasiddha Krishnacharya, also known [to Tibetans] as Lobpon Acharyapa (Tib. sLob dpon a tsar ya pa). Here these previously existent oral traditions are used as the basis. This is enriched and clarified in reference to *The Sambhuta Drop of Springtime* (Skt. *Samputa tilaka*) and also Acharya Krishnacharya's *The Drop of Springtime* (Skt. *Vasanta tilaka*).

The illusory body and the clear light doctrines are derived from the Guhyasamaja oral tradition, as taught by the Indian mahasiddha Jnanagarbha and received [by Marpa directly from him]. Thus these are based on the Guhyasamaja Tantra. Here the Marpa tradition of the Guhyasamaja oral instruction transmission has been used as the basis, with references to the Guhyasamaja cycle of the Aryas, Father and Sons [i.e., "The Arya Cycle of Guhyasamaja Doctrines"].

The practices of consciousness transference and forceful projection to a new residence are based on the Four Seats Tantra. In addition, one should understand that they are associated with numerous other tantric traditions, including the Sambhuta Tantra, the Vajradaka Tantra, and so forth. I have explained these two in a manner affording easy understanding. As these teachings are based on these reliable sources, one should have confidence in them.

> Oh hark!
> The incomparable Buddha Shakyamuni, lord of sages,
> Taught the holy Dharma for the benefit of living beings.
> Supreme of his teachings are those of highest yoga tantra,
> Both the female tantras and the male tantras.
>
> From the female tantras [i.e., Hevajra and Chakrasamvara]
> Comes the teaching on the inner heat doctrine, *chandali*,
> A method for bringing the subtle energies under control
> And arousing the innate wisdom.
>
> With this as the basis one takes up the practice
> Of the illusory body and clear light doctrines
> That emanate from the Guhyasamaja Tantra,
> And the doctrines of consciousness transference
> And forceful projection to another residence
> That emanate from the Shri Chaturpitha Tantra.
>
> Based on those sources there arose
> This tradition from the mahasiddhas Tilopa and Naropa,
> Famed as "the Six Yogas of Naropa."

Countless practitioners here in this land of snows
Have delighted in this festival of profound tantric endeavor,
A deeply cherished and precious oral tradition legacy.

By the force of great merits from previous lives,
Miwang Drakpa became famed throughout this domain
As a chieftain dedicated to the Six Yogas tradition;
He wears the Three Jewels as his crown ornaments.
And Chojey Sonam, whose wisdom pulsates
With having read the sacred scriptures in depth, and who
Has become rich in profound spiritual realization.
These two offered me a mandala decorated with jewels
And requested me to write this treatise.
Moreover, these days there are many practitioners
With great interest in this sublime path;
Therefore, thinking that it may be of benefit to some,
I made the effort and composed this work.

It contains clear instructions on the stages of meditation in this
    path,
A clear and critical guide to the principles in the trainings,
And references to the authoritative tantras and commentaries;
These are the three features within which it is set.

The essential meanings of the profound teachings are hard to
    perceive
And ordinary beings cannot easily penetrate them.
Hence I request the dakas and dakinis
To be patient with any faults [of the book].

Through any merits resulting from this composition,
May all beings enter into peerless tantric practice;
And may this sublime tradition [known as the Six Yogas of
    Naropa] prosper and grow.

The Colophon

This treatise on the profound path of the Six Yogas of Naropa, entitled *A Book of Three Inspirations*, was written at the repeated requests
of the lordly Miwang Drakpa Gyaltsen and Chojey Sonam Gyaltsen,
who asked for a work that would clarify the key points in the inner
heat yogas, as well as briefly touch upon the common and exclusive
distinctions in the trainings.[61]

Even though this tradition has inspired extraordinary activities
in this part of the world over the past generations, these days the

practice of it is not particularly widespread. Yet there are many people with interest in it, and therefore I thought that perhaps it may be useful to accept the request.

It was composed by a Buddhist monk who had heard many teachings, Lobzang Drakpa of the East, while residing in Ganden Namgyal Ling Monastery on Nomad Mountain. The scribe was Kazhipa Rinchen Pal.

May goodness increase in the world.

APPENDIX I

Vajrasattva Meditation and Mantra Recitation

from Tsongkhapa's *A Book of Three Inspirations*

One begins the meditation session by blending deeply into one's mindstream thoughts of the Three Jewels of Refuge, until a strong sense of refuge arises. Then one thinks to oneself, "Just as I myself am drowning in the ocean of samsara, so are all other sentient beings. Moreover, all of them have been a mother to me in many of my previous lives, and on those occasions showed me great kindness, benefiting me in countless ways and protecting me from harm."

Reflect in this way, and give rise to a consistent attitude to repay all sentient beings for the kindnesses they have thus shown to you.

Next contemplate the ways in which sentient beings are deprived of happiness and are afflicted with suffering. Give rise to the strong aspiration to establish them in every happiness and to free them from every suffering.

Then one asks oneself, "And just who has the ability to completely accomplish these two aims?" The answer is that only a completely enlightened being, a buddha, can do so.

One meditates like this until a strong sense of the bodhimind arises, which is the experience of universal responsibility that aspires to accomplish buddhahood as a means of benefiting all living beings.

Like that, one should repeatedly stabilize the decision to rely upon the path by thinking that one must accomplish enlightenment for the benefit of all living beings.

The Essential Ornament (Skt. *Hridaya alamkara*) states,

> The embodiment of all the buddhas
> Appears upon seats of a white lotus and moon
> As Vajrasattva, adorned with vajra, bell and ornaments.
> Visualize in this way.

> The hundred-syllable mantra is recited twenty-one times.
> Through the blessing power of this recitation,
> The karmic stains of failings are cleansed
> And the increasing power of negative karma will not manifest.

> This has been said by the mahasiddhas.
> Also, practice this mantra between yoga sessions;
> And if one can complete 100,000 mantra recitations,
> One will become in nature utterly purified.

As said above, if one relies upon the meditation and mantra recitation focusing upon Vajrasattva, repeating the hundred-syllable Vajrasattva mantra twenty-one times [at the beginning of each yoga session], the increasing power of negative karmic forces created by spiritual failings and so forth will no longer be able to manifest and multiply.

Moreover, if one can recite the hundred-syllable mantra 100,000 times, one will accomplish utter purification of all spiritual faults. This has been said by many great masters of the past.

Therefore, one should undertake this practice with confidence. As the Vajrasattva meditation and mantra recitation fulfills such sublime purposes, one should engage in it with enthusiasm.

The visualization to be pursued is as follows.

Upon one's head appears a white syllable *PAM*. This becomes a white lotus, with a syllable *AH* resting above it. This syllable transforms into a moon disk, the syllable *HUM* resting above it. *HUM* transforms into a white, five-pronged vajra, with a syllable *HUM* marking its center.

Lights go out from this, accomplish the two purposes [of oneself and others], and then are reabsorbed [into the vajra and *HUM*]. This utterly transforms, and Vajrasattva instantly appears [upon the lotus and moon seats], his body white in color, holding a vajra in his right hand and a bell in his left, the consort white Vajra Bhagavati embracing him, her hands holding a curved knife and a cup made of a human skull.

He is adorned by the precious ornaments, and his body possesses the marks and signs of perfection. He is seated in the vajra posture [i.e., legs folded over one another], and a white syllable *HUM* stands upon a moon disk at his heart. [This is the Samayasattva, or Symbolic Being.]

Lights emanate forth from the *HUM* at his heart, summoning forth the Jnanasattvas, or Wisdom Beings. They appear in the same form as he. One makes devotional offerings to them and recites the mantra *JAH HUM BAM HOH*, summoning them to, dissolving them into, merging them with and making them inseparable from him.

Again lights are sent forth from the syllable *HUM* at his heart. They summon the Initiation Deities. One makes devotional offerings to them, and requests them, "O Tathagatas, You Gone to Suchness, please bestow empowerment."

The Tathagatas think to bestow empowerment. Their consorts hold up jewelled vases filled with wisdom empowerment nectars, and sing the auspicious verse,

> Just as at the time of the Buddha's birth
> Celestial beings appeared and bathed him,
> So do we bathe you now
> With these mystical empowerment nectars.
> *OM SARVA TATHAGATA ABHISHEKATA SAMAYA SHRI YA HUM*

Saying this, they pour forth wisdom nectars from their vases. The body [of Vajrasattva visualized above the crown of one's head], is filled. Buddha Akshobya appears as [Vajrasattva's] crown ornament.

One now assumes a devotional posture of body, speech and mind, and makes the request, "O Bhagavan Vajrasattva, please bless me to purify all negative karmic seeds, spiritual obscurations, and degenerated precepts accumulated by myself and others."

When this supplication has been made, lights emanate forth from the syllable *HUM* at his heart. They touch all living beings, purifying them of negative karmic instincts, spiritual obscurations, and weakening of precepts.

The lights then make devotional offerings to the buddhas and bodhisattvas of the ten directions, which cause the transformative energies of body, speech, mind, realizations and activity power of all enlightened beings to manifest as light. This light then flows into the syllable HUM at Vajrasattva's heart. One contemplates that in this way [the visualized] Vajrasattva becomes brilliantly radiant and imbued with every perfection and power.

One now concentrates on the HUM at Vajrasattva's heart. It is encircled by the hundred-syllable mantra:

> OM VAJRA HERUKA SAMAYA / MANUPALAYA / HERUKA
> TVENOTAPISHTHA / DRIDHO MEBHAVA / SUTOSHYO MEBHAVA /
> SUPOSHYO MEBHAVA / ANURAKTO MEBHAVA / SARVA SIDDHI
> MEPRAYACHHA / SARVA KARMA SUCHAME / CHHITAM SHRI YAM
> / KURU HUM/ HA HA HA HA HOH BHAGAVAN / VAJRA HERUKA
> MAME MUCHA / HERUKA BHAVA / MAHA SAMAYA SATTVA AH
> HUM PHAT

One visualizes the hundred-syllable mantra as surrounding the seed syllable [HUM] in this way. Lights emanate from the mantric syllables, purify living beings of negative karmic instincts and spiritual obscurations, and make inconceivably vast offerings to the buddhas and bodhisattvas. The transformative blessing powers of the body, speech and mind of the buddhas and bodhisattvas are drawn forth, and are absorbed into the mantric syllables.

A stream of white nectars flows forth from the mantric seeds. They flow downward, and exit the bodies of Vajrasattva and Consort from the place of their sexual union. They come to the crown of one's head, where they flow into one's body via the Brahma aperture. All negative karmic instincts and obscurations collected by means of activities of body, speech and mind are expelled, and are visualized as leaving one's body via the bodily apertures and pores, in the form of thick black slime. One is purified of all negative karma and obscurations, and one's body becomes filled with a radiantly white stream of wisdom nectars. Both oneself and all other living beings are infused with every spiritual knowledge and excellence. Meditate in this way as you recite the mantra.

At the conclusion of the meditation session apply the four purification forces (such as acknowledging one's shortcomings and failings, generating remorse at one's failures, and so forth). Then contemplate the non-truly-existent, voidness nature of the three circles of negative karma and obscurations: how the negative karma and obscurations themselves, oneself as the perpetrator and experiencer of them, and the act of perpetrating and experiencing them, all have no real or inherent existence. Conclude the meditation session with the verse,

> I, confused by unknowing,
> May have transgressed the precepts.
> O guru, great protector, inspire me.
> Especially, O Buddha Vajrasattva,
> Whose nature is great compassion,
> Lord of living beings, grant refuge.

Vajrasattva replies, "Child of good character, your negative karmic instincts, spiritual obscurations and failures in training are all now purified."

Having said this, he dissolves into one's body. Meditate that in this way one's body, speech and mind become inseparable from the body, speech and mind of Vajrasattva.

Conclude the session by dedicating the merit of the practice and offering auspicious prayers.

APPENDIX II

Establishing Blessing Powers by Meditating upon Guru Yoga

from Tsongkhapa's *A Book of Three Inspirations*

This is explained under two headings: meditating upon the guru as a field of merit; and offering devotions and prayers.

The first of these is done as follows. One visualizes that in the space in front of oneself is a jeweled throne supported by lions. It bears a seat made of a lotus and a sun disk. Upon that sits one's own guru. In nature he is one's guru, but in appearance he resembles Buddha Vajradhara, lord of the sixth buddha family, his body blue in color. His two hands, with a vajra in the right and a bell in the left, embrace a consort who resembles him. His upper and lower robes are made of celestial silks, and he is adorned with the jewel ornaments. His legs are crossed in the vajra posture, and he is ablaze with the lights of five colors.

Meditating in this way, envision that at his crown chakra the white syllable *OM* rests upon a moon disk; at his throat chakra the red syllable *AH* rests upon a lotus; and at his heart chakra the blue syllable *HUM* rests upon a sun disk. All three syllables are ablaze with lights.

A great radiance emanates forth from the syllable *HUM*, summoning forth Buddha Vajradhara, the assembly of lineage gurus, and the host of meditational mandala deities. They all dissolve into the Buddha Vajradhara visualized in front.

As is said in *The Arising of Samvara Tantra,*

> The guru is the Buddha, the guru is the Dharma,
> And likewise the guru is the Sangha.

In this way meditate that the guru is the embodiment of all Three
Jewels of Refuge.

Also *The Five Stages* states,

> The self-realized Buddha
> Is a singularly super divinity.
> But one's own tantric master is even greater,
> For it is he or she who gives one the oral transmissions.

As said above, one should think that the guru who is one's personal
field of merit and who gives one the tantric teachings is even greater
than Buddha Vajradhara himself.

Also, *The Book of Manjushri's Direct Instruction* states,

> In sum, when the meaningful is being undertaken,
> I shall reside within that body.
> Thus another shall accept the devotion of the practice.
> By that devotion and the joy it produces,
> Karmic obscurations will be purified from the mindstream.

As said here, sometimes when teacher and disciples gather for the
purpose of transmitting the oral traditions, the buddhas themselves
come, enter into the teacher's body, and accept the devotion themselves. This spontaneously gives rise to great joy in the minds of the
disciples.

When on other occasions one practices devotion [i.e., when not in
the presence of the guru], although one gains the merit of offering
devotion to the buddhas, it is not as sure that the buddhas will manifest to accept it directly, and thus the level of the merit is not as certain. Thus one can have confidence that the guru is the unsurpassed
field of merit.

Hence one should regard the guru as an embodiment of all the
Tathagatas. Resolve to transcend the mind that sees faults in the guru,
and cultivate the habit of appreciating the guru's realizations. From
within this sphere of awareness, engage in acts of devotion.

If one relates to the guru on the basis of looking for faults in him or
her, one merely creates obstacles to the accomplishment of the siddhis.
Conversely, if one relates to the spiritual master on the basis of looking for his or her realizations, one quickly achieves the siddhis.

Therefore one should cultivate the ways of relating to the guru on the basis of positive energy, being mindful of his or her kindness, and treating him or her with great respect.

OFFERING DEVOTIONS AND PRAYERS

The Five Stages states,

> Leave behind all ordinary devotion
> And take up devotion to the guru;
> For by pleasing the guru one attains
> The supreme wisdom of omniscient buddhahood.
>
> Devoting oneself to the master who teaches highest tantra
> While seeing him as a tantric buddha in human form:
> What is the limit of the merit thus accrued?
> What path is there that is less austere?

As said here, the supreme devotion is devotion to the guru. Generate intense awareness of this dynamic, and devote yourself accordingly to your tantric teacher.

One such devotional exercise is that of offering the mandala symbolic of the universe.

Here one takes a base made of anything from simple clay to the most ornate jewelled materials, and consecrates it with blessed cow products, perfumed waters, and the five nectars. One begins with the mantra OM VAJRA BHUMI AH HUM, and while saying it, pours flower petals (or whatever substances are being used, such as grains, sand, jewels, etc.) over the base, while reciting, "Here is the great powerful golden earth."

Then with the mantra OM VAJRA REKHE AH HUM one pours more flower petals, this time in a circle around the outer circumference of the base, while reciting, "Here is the surrounding iron fence." Next one takes a handful of flower petals consecrated with perfumes and the five nectars, and pours them into the center of the base, reciting, "and here is the great Mount Meru."

One then pours a handful of flower petals successively into the eastern, southern, western and northern directions, while reciting, "In the east is the continent Lupakpo, in the south Jambuling, in the west Balangcho, and in the north Draminyan."

Now one places a handful to the right and left of each of these continents in order to symbolize the subcontinents, beginning with the east and moving clockwise as above. Thus one does so with the

eastern continent, while reciting the names of the two eastern subcontinents Lu and Lupak; then to the right and left of the southern
continent, Ngayab and Ngayabzhan; next to the right and left of the
western continent while reciting "Yodan and Lamchokdro"; and to
the right and left of the northern continent while reciting "Draminyan
and Draminyan Kyida."

Then one pours a handful on top of the continents, first to the east,
reciting "the precious elephant"; then above the south while reciting
"the precious lord"; above the west while reciting "the precious supreme horse"; above the north while reciting "the precious queen";
above the southeast while reciting "the precious warrior"; above the
southwest while reciting "the precious wheel"; above the northwest
while reciting "the precious jewel"; and above the northeast while
reciting "the precious treasure." Then to the east of the center one
pours a handful of flowers, reciting, "the sun"; and to the west of the
center, reciting, "the moon."

In this way one creates a symbolic universe with all auspicious
things in it, visualizing it as being made of various precious gems.
One holds it up and offers it to the guru, while reciting the following
words: "I send forth as an offering in the manner exemplified by the
great bodhisattva Samantabhadra this symbolic universe made of
precious gems, together with the mass of meritorious energy collected
in the past, present and future by myself and all other living beings
through our actions of body, speech and mind. All of this I envision
within my mind and offer to my gurus, meditational deities, and the
forces of spiritual refuge. Accept it out of your compassion, and bestow waves of inspiring power upon me."

Thus one offers the mandala to the guru. Here the flower petals (or
whatever substances) that are used are the outer offering; and the
five nectars with which these are anointed are the inner offering. One
should also make the secret offering, chant verses of praise, and in
the presence of the visualized assembly renew whatever general and
particular pledges of practice one has previously adopted.

Then with great reverence one should chant several prayers re-
questing blessings to inspire one to quickly generate within one's
mindstream the realizations of the actual experience of the stages of
the ordinary [i.e., general Mahayana] and extraordinary [i.e.,
Vajrayana] paths, as well as to pacify adverse conditions and create
conducive conditions to accomplishing these stages of realization.

The guru is pleased at one's efforts. From his three points [i.e., forehead, throat and heart] respectively emanate forth white, red and blue lights. These enter into one's own three points, and one's body becomes completely filled with them. One is purified of all negative karmic seeds that were collected by means of body, speech and mind, and receives the first three empowerments, known by the names "vase," "secret" and "wisdom awareness." The three realizations—those of vajra body, vajra speech and vajra mind—successively are induced. One meditates in this way.

Now a great mass of multicolored lights emanate from all [three] sites of the guru's body. They enter one's body via all [three] of one's sites. The most subtle obscurations generated by means of body, speech and mind are simultaneously purified. One receives the fourth empowerment, known as "the initiation of highest significance." The realizations of the inseparable three vajras are induced.

Here the three mantric syllables symbolize the three vajras [i.e., the perfected states of body, speech and mind]. Just as the lights from these syllables are visualized as purifying the obscurations of body, speech and mind, the empowerments known as vase, secret and wisdom awareness purify these three types of karmic stains. Similarly the fourth empowerment, known as "the empowerment of highest significance," purifies the obscurations to realizing the inseparable nature of the three vajras.

The process explained above is merely a symbolic method of achieving the four empowerments, and not the actual obtaining of the empowerments.

One then brings the guru visualized in front to the space above one's head, either by mantra and mudra, or else simply by visualizing the process. He or she then dissolves into one's body, and one meditates that one's body, speech and mind become inseparable in nature from the holy body, speech and mind of the guru. One recites the hundred syllable mantra [of Vajrasattva, as outlined earlier].

This practice should be done between yoga sessions, and at the beginning of each session.

GLOSSARY

Sanskrit and Tibetan Names and Terms

<table>
<tr><td colspan="2" align="center">SANSKRIT</td></tr>
<tr><td>Abhidharma</td><td>Abhidharma</td></tr>
<tr><td>abhisheka</td><td>abhiṣeka</td></tr>
<tr><td>acharya</td><td>ācārya</td></tr>
<tr><td>Acharya Vira</td><td>Ācārya Vira</td></tr>
<tr><td>Adibuddha</td><td>adibuddha</td></tr>
<tr><td>Akanishta</td><td>Akaniṣṭha</td></tr>
<tr><td>Akshobhya</td><td>Akṣobhya</td></tr>
<tr><td>Amitayus</td><td>Amitāyus</td></tr>
<tr><td>anuttara yoga tantra</td><td>anuttarayogatantra</td></tr>
<tr><td>arhat</td><td>arhat</td></tr>
<tr><td>arya</td><td>ārya</td></tr>
<tr><td>Aryashura</td><td>Āryaśūra</td></tr>
<tr><td>Asanga</td><td>Asaṅga</td></tr>
<tr><td>Ashvaghosha</td><td>Aśvaghoṣa</td></tr>
<tr><td>Atisha</td><td>Atiśa</td></tr>
<tr><td>avadhuti</td><td>avadhūti</td></tr>
<tr><td>ayatana</td><td>āyatana</td></tr>
<tr><td>bhagavan</td><td>bhagavan</td></tr>
<tr><td>Bhavabhadra</td><td>Bhavabhadra</td></tr>
<tr><td>bindu</td><td>bindu</td></tr>
<tr><td>bodhichitta</td><td>bodhicitta</td></tr>
<tr><td>bodhisattva</td><td>bodhisattva</td></tr>
<tr><td>Bodhisattvayana</td><td>Bodhisattvayāna</td></tr>
<tr><td>Buddha</td><td>Buddha</td></tr>
</table>

chakra	cakra
Chakrasamvara	Cakrasaṃvara
chandali	caṇḍālī
Chandrakirti	Candrakīrti
charya	caryā
daka	ḍāka
dakini	ḍākinī
Dharma	dharma
Dharmabhadra	Dharmabhadra
Dharmakaya	Dharmakāya
Dharmapala	dharmapāla
dharmata	dharmatā
dhatu	dhātu
dhuti	dhuti
dhyana	dhyāna
Dipamkara Shrijnana	Dīpaṃkara Śrījñāna
Dombipada	Ḍombīpāda
Ghantapada	Ghaṇṭāpāda
Guhyasamaja	Guhyasamāja
Hayagriva	Hayagrīva
Heruka	Heruka
Hevajra	Hevajra
Hinayana	Hinayāna
Jnanabhadra	Jñānabhadra
Jnanagarbha	Jñānagarbha
jnanamudra	jñānamudrā
Jnanasattva	jñānasattva
Kalachakra	Kālacakra
kamadhatu	kāmadhātu
karmamudra	karmamudrā
kaya	kāya
klesha	kleśa
klesha avarana	kleśāvaraṇa
Krishnacharya	Kṛṣṇācārya
kriya	kriyā
lalana	lalanā
Lawapa	Lva va pā
Luipa	Lūipā
Madhyamaka	Madhyamaka
Madhyamika	Mādhyamika
Mahamaya	Mahāmāyā
maha anuttara yoga tantra	mahānuttarayogatantra
mahamudra	mahāmudrā
mahasiddha	mahāsiddha
Mahasukhakaya	Mahāsukhakāya
Mahayana	Mahāyāna

Maitreya	Maitreya
Maitripa	Maitrīpa
mandala	maṇḍala
Manjushri	Mañjuśrī
Mantrayana	Mantrayāna
mudra	mudrā
mulatantra	mūlatantra
nada	nāḍa
nadi	nāḍī
Nagarjuna	Nāgārjuna
Nairatmya	Nairātmyā
Nalanda	Nālandā
Naro	Nāro
Naropa	Nāropā
Nirmanakaya	Nirmāṇakāya
Padma	Padma
Padmasambhava	Padmasaṃbhava
pandita	paṇḍita
paramita	pāramitā
Paramitayana	Pāramitāyāna
prajna	prajñā
Prajnaparamita	Prajñāpāramitā
prana	prāṇa
rasana	rasanā
rupadhatu	rūpadhātu
rupakaya	rūpakāya
sadhana	sādhana
Sahajavajra	Sahajavajra
samadhi	samādhi
samaya	samaya
samayamudra	samayamudrā
Samayasattva	Samayasattva
Samayavajra	Samayavajra
Sambhogakaya	Sambhogakāya
Sambhuta	Sambhūta
samsara	saṃsāra
Sangha	Saṅgha
Sautrantika	Sautrāntika
Shakyamuni	Śākyamuni
shamata	śamatha
Shantideva	Śāntideva
shastra	śāstra
Shravaka	Śrāvaka
Shravakayana	Śrāvakayāna
shunyata	śūnyatā
siddha	siddha

Siddharani	Siddharāṇi
siddhi	siddhi
skandha	skandha
Sukhavati	Sukhāvatī
Sukhasiddhi	Sukhasiddhi
sutra	sūtra
Sutrayana	Sūtrayāna
tantra	tantra
Tantrayana	Tantrayāna
Tathagata	Tathāgata
Tulakshetra	Tulakṣetra
Tushita	Tuṣita
Uttara tantra yana	Uttaratantrayāna
Vaibhashika	Vaibhāṣika
vajra	vajra
Vajra Bhagavati	Vajra Bhagavatī
Vajrabhairava	Vajrabhairava
Vajradaka	Vajraḍāka
Vajradhara	Vajradhara
Vajrasattva	Vajrasattva
Vajrayana	Vajrayāna
Vajrayogini	Vajrayoginī
Vasubandhu	Vasubandhu
vayu	vāyu
Vijnanavadin	Vijñānavādin
Vikramashila	Vikramaśila
vipasyana	vipaśyanā
Yamantaka	Yamāntaka
yana	yāna
Yogachara	Yogācāra
yuganaddha	yuganaddha

TIBETAN

AH tung	a thung
bardo	bar do
Bari Lotsawa	Ba ri lo tsā ba
Basowa Tenpai Gyaltsen	Ba so ba bsTan pa'i rgyal mtshan
Bodong Chokley Namgyal	Bo dong Phyogs las rnam rgyal
Bonpo	Bon po
Buton Rinchen Drup	Bu ston Rin chen sgrub
Chak Lotsawa	Chag lo tsa ba
Chiterpa	sPyi ter pa
Chojey Sonam Gyaltsen	Chos rje bSod nams rgyal mtshan
Chojey Gampopa	Chos rje sGam po pa

Chokro	Cok ro
Chokyi Dorjey	Chos kyi rdo rje
Damchoe Gyaltsen	Dam chos rgyal mtshan
Darma Dodey	Dar ma mdo sde
Dolma Podrang	sGrol ma pho drang
Drakpa Jangchup	Grags pa byang chub
Drikung	'Bri gung
Drikung Jigten Gonpo	'Bri gung 'Jig rten dgon po
Drikung Kargyupa	'Bri gung bka' brgyud pa
Drukpa Kargyupa	'Brug pa bka' brgyud pa
Dakpo	Dvags po
Gampopa	sGam po pa
Ganden	dGa' ldan
Ganden Shartsey	dGa' ldan shar rtse
Gandenpa	dGa' ldan pa
Geluk	dGe lugs
Gelukpa	dGe lugs pa
Gendun Chopel	dGe bdun chos 'phel
Goe Lotsawa	'Gos lo tsā ba
gyalpo	rGyal po
Gyaltsab Jey	rGyal tshab rje
Gyalwa	rGyal ba
Gyalwa Nyipa	rGyal ba gnyis pa
Jampa Palwa	Byams pa dpal ba
Jetsun	rJe btsun
Jey Gyalwa Nyipa	rJe rgyal ba gnyis pa
Jey Sherab Gyatso	rJe shes rab rgya mtsho
Jigten Gonpo	'Jig rten dgon po
Jigten Sumgon	'Jig rten gsum dgon
Jonangpa	Jo nang pa
Kadam	bKa' gdams
Kadampa	bKa' gdams pa
Kajou Zhing	mKha' spyod zhing
Kargyu	bKa' brgyud
Kargyupa	bKa' brgyud pa
Karma Tashi Namgyal	Kar ma bkra shis rnam rgyal
Karmapa	Kar ma pa
Kham	Khams
Khedrup Jampa Pel	mKhas grub byams pa dpal
Khedrup Jey	mKhas grub rje
Khedrup Gelek Palzangpo	mKhas grub dge legs dpal bzang po
Lawapa	La bva pa
ley kor	klad kor
Lhasa	lHa sa
Lobpon	Slob dpon
Lobzang Chogyen	Blo bzang chos rgyan

Lobzang Drakpa	Blo bzang grags pa
Lochen Rinchen Zangpo	Lo chen Rin chen bzang po
Lochung	lHo brag
Lodrak	Lo chung
Lotsawa	Lo tsa ba
Luipa	Lu'i pa
Maitripa	Mee tri pa
Mardo	Mar do
Marpa	Mar pa
Marpa Lotsawa	Mar pa lo tsa ba
Maryul	Mar yul
Maryul Loden	Mar yul blo ldan
Menkangpa	sMan khang pa
menngak	Man ngag
Mey	Mes
Meyton	Mes ston
Meytson	Mes tshon
Milarepa	Mi la ras pa
Miwang Drakpa Gyaltsen	Mi dbang grags pa rgyal mtshan
Monlam Chenmo	sMon lam chen mo
Namgyal Ling	rNam rgyal gling
Ngawang Palden	Ngag dbang dpal ldan
Ngok	rNgog
Ngok Lekpai Sherab	rNgog Legs pa'i shes rab
Ngokton	rNgog ston
Ngulchu Dharmabhadra	dNgul chu Dhar ma bha dra
Nyingma	rNying ma
Nyingmapa	rNying ma pa
Olkha	dBol kha
Pabongkha Dechen Nyingpo	Pha bong kha bDe chen snying po
Pakmo Drupa	dPal phag mo gru pa
Pema Karpo	Pad ma dkar po
Puntsok Podrang	Phun tshogs pho drang
rang luk	Rang lugs
Rechungpa	Ras chung pa
Rinpochey	Rin po che
Sakya	Sa skya
Sakyapa	Sa skya pa
Sangyey Yeshey	Sang rgyas ye shes
Sempa Chenpo Kunzangpa	Sems dpa' chen po Kun bzang pa
Sonam Gyaltsen	bSod nams rgyal mtshan
Sonam Sengey	bSod nams seng ge
Sonam Wangpo	bSod nams dbang po
Tilbupa	Dril bu pa
Tipupa	Ti phu pa

torma	gTor ma
Trizur Ngawang Chokden	'Khrid zur Ngag dbang mchog ldan
Tsang	gTsang
Tsangpa Rechung	gTsang pa ras chung
tsig bu	tsig bu
Tsongkhapa Chenpo	Tsong kha pa chen po
Tsur	'Tshur
Tsurton	'Tshur ston
tummo	gTum mo
Wensapa Lobzang Dondup	dBen sa pa blo bzang don grub
Yangonpa	Yang dgon pa
yidam	Yi dam
Yongdzin Pandita	Yongs 'dzin pan di ta
Zangkar	Zangs dkar
Zhalu	Zha lu

Notes

Introduction

1. *Sutras, tantras* and *shastras*: The first of these refers to the open discourses of the Buddha, which, with the exception of the *Vinaya sutra*, were transmitted orally for several centuries before being written down. The second refers to the esoteric teachings given by the Buddha in mystical states. The third refers to the treatises and commentaries composed by later Indian masters.

The first two categories of scriptures are contained in the Tibetan canonical collection known as the *Kangyur* (Tib. bKa' 'gyur); the third comprises the Tibetan canonical collection known as the *Tangyur* (bsTan 'gyur).

2. The Three Great Dharma Kings: Songtsen Gampo (Tib. Srong btsan sgam po), who in the mid-seventh century made Buddhism the national religion of Tibet; Trisong Deutsen (Tib. Khri srong deu btsan), who in the mid-eighth century brought Guru Padmasambhava to Tibet and established the country's first full-fledged monastery, in addition to overseeing much translation work; and, half a century later, Tri Ralpachen (Khri Ral pa can), who patronized the systematic overhaul and standardization of all earlier translations, thus completing the work of the first two.

All three of these Great Dharma Kings are considered to be previous incarnations of the being who was to become the First Dalai Lama.

3. There is a tendency these days to speak of the Nyingma as though it were one school; prior to 1959 most Nyingma monasteries were independent, and there was never one "head lama" of the Nyingmapa, as opposed to the New Schools, each of which had its own patriarch. Each of the twelve Kargyupa schools, for example, had its own head lama.

4. Goe Lotsawa's (Tib. 'Gos lo tsa wa) *The Blue Annals* (Tib. *Deb ther sngon po*), translated by George Roerich with the assistance of Gendun Chopel (Calcutta, 1949), presents the most historically accurate analysis of the life of Marpa available in English. However, *The Life of Marpa the Translator* (Boulder: Prajna,

1982), prepared by the meticulous Nalanda Translation Committee under the direction of Chogyam Trungpa from the sixteenth-century Tibetan text of Tsangnyon Heruka (Tib. Tsangs snyon he ru ka; b. 1452), provides a more romanticized and more readable account. Tsangnyon's work is hagiography, and thus is more concerned with providing an inspiring story than with historical precision.

This latter text portrays Marpa as having been sent by Naropa to study with Jnanagarbha, Maitripa and the mahasiddha Kukuripa. Goe Lotsawa does not confirm this, and instead suggests he met his other masters quite independently of Naropa.

The translators of *The Blue Annals* imply that Jnanagarbha and Kukuripa are in fact one and the same person (page 400).

5. One usually sees the group names of these four older and eight younger Kargyupa sub-sects translated as "four greater" and "eight lesser." Although the Tibetan terms *che* and *chung* can sometimes have this meaning, usually they do not. In this context translating them as "great" and "small" is distinctly misleading. For instance, the Drikung Kargyu, one of the eight younger schools, was probably larger than all four older schools combined. In fact, two of the four older sects barely survived into the twentieth century.

6. For a discussion of his importance to the Tibetan understanding of the Kalachakra tantric tradition, see my *The Practice of Kalachakra* (Ithaca: Snow Lion Publications, 1991).

7. Herbert Guenther's *The Life and Teachings of Naropa* (London: Oxford University Press, 1963) is based on his translation of the Tibetan biography composed by Lhatsun Rinchen Namgyal (Tib. lHa btsun rin chen rnam rgyal), a direct disciple of Tsangnyon Heruka, the author of the biography of Marpa mentioned in note 4 above. It is in the same genre, and aims more at providing exciting and inspirational reading rather than giving "factual" history. This adds to its charm rather than detracts from it.

8. No major biography of Tilopa has been translated, although small accounts are given in several sources. My favorite is to be found in *The Great Kagyu Masters* by Khenpo Konchög Gyaltsen (Ithaca: Snow Lion Publications, 1990).

9. See *Selected Works of the Dalai Lama II: The Tantric Yogas of Sister Niguma* (Ithaca: Snow Lion Publications, 1984).

10. It is interesting that Tsongkhapa does not elaborate on the *Vajra Song of the Six Yogas*, which he mentions in his Epilogue and to which Jey Sherab Gyatso referred in the quotation given on page 22. I am not sure exactly what text this is. It may be Tilopa's *Oral Instruction on the Six Doctrines* (Tib. *Chos drug gi man ngag*) and I have listed it as such in the bibliography. However, it also could refer to Naropa's *Whispered Instruction of the Six Dharmas* (Tib. *Chos drug snyan rgyud*), which is not included in the Peking Tangyur but is to be found in the Dergey Tangyur. Tsongkhapa mentions the title only as *The Vajra Song of the Six Yogas* (*Chos drug rdo rje mgur*), and there is no direct equivalent of this. Moreover, he

does not quote or discuss the text, other than saying that it is "only intended to plant the seeds of the oral tradition teaching" and also that it is "too terse to do much more than that." I include both Tilopa's and Naropa's texts in *Readings on the Six Yogas of Naropa* (Ithaca: Snow Lion Publications, forthcoming).

11. Translated in my study of the Thirteenth's life and teachings, *Path of the Bodhisattva Warrior* (Ithaca: Snow Lion Publications, 1988).

12. Tenzin Gyatso, His Holiness the Dalai Lama, *Cultivating a Daily Meditation* (Dharamsala: Library of Tibetan Works and Archives, 1991).

13. Unfortunately Pema Karpo does not describe the more extensive numbers of the physical exercises, such as the twenty or fifty, nor give a literary source for them. See *Tibetan Yoga and Secret Doctrines*, translated by Lama Kazi Dawa-Samdup and W. Y. Evans-Wentz (London: Oxford University Press, 1935), p.207.

14. *Tummo*, or inner heat (Skt. *chandali*; Tib. *gtum mo*) is rendered by several modern translators as "the Fierce Woman." Although *mo* is a female suffix and *gtum* has a sense of both fierceness and heat about it, the English words "fierce woman" would most directly be re-translated back into Tibetan as *kyemen drakpo* (Tib. *skyes dman drag po*), and if presented to any Tibetan lama as an equivalent of *tummo* would certainly bring a chuckle from his lips. It is a bit like translating the French *la table* as Miss Flat-top.

There is, of course, a tradition of representing the different chakras by dakinis. Similarly, in the body mandala practices of the Chakrasamvara systems one visualizes tantric deities at each of the main bodily sites, the various bodily energies are symbolized by deities, and so forth.

15. I use this translation of the Tibetan term *a thung* (literally "the short *AH*") as a tribute to the late Chogyam Trungpa Rinpochey, who used it in his work on the life of Marpa mentioned above. For all his eccentricities and the tragic end to his life—he died of alcoholism—Trungpa was one of the great lamas of our time in terms of communicating the essential sense of Tibetan Buddhism to Western culture.

16. Dr. Herbert Benson's research with Tibetan yogis is partially documented in his book *Beyond the Relaxation Response* (New York: Times Books, 1984). A video of his project was also made.

17. I say this because it was evident at a discourse I attended on the various mudra practices in 1974 from a highly qualified and traditional Gelukpa monk. An Italian monk asked, "Does a monk who wishes to practice karmamudra have to disrobe in order to do so?" The lama laughed and replied, "No. He just becomes an especially good monk."

18. The First Dalai Lama's treatise, *Notes on the Two Yogic Stages of Glorious Kalachakra* (Tib. *dPal dus kyi 'khor lo'i rim pa gnyis pa'i zin bris*), is translated in my book on the Kalachakra tantric system, *The Practice of Kalachakra* (Ithaca: Snow Lion Publications, 1991), which includes translations of eight different Tibetan texts on various aspects of the Kalachakra tradition.

19. Abhidharma is one of the three classes of Sutrayana literature: Sutra, Abhidharma and Vinaya. The first of these mainly deals with meditation, the second with metaphysics, and the third with philosophy of ethics. All of Buddha's teachings in the Sutrayana classification belong to one of these three divisions.

Tibetans generally study the Abhidharma teachings based on the shastras, or treatises of the later Indian masters, which extract the essence of the Buddha's words as recorded in the diverse sources and present them thematically. Their two favorite Abhidharma shastras are the *Abhidharma kosha* of Vasubandhu and the *Abhidharma samucchaya* of Asanga.

20. *Tibetan Yoga and Secret Doctrines*, a collection of esoteric tantric texts translated from the Tibetan by Lama Kazi Dawa-Samdup and W. Y. Evans-Wentz (London: Oxford University Press, 1935), was one of the first English language publications to present a complete and reliable discussion of the Six Yogas of Naropa. The translations do contain some minor errors due to the limitations of the two translators and the conditions under which the work was done, but sixty years later still stand as excellent portraits of various aspects of Tibetan tantric meditation and yoga.

21. I discuss these in chapter seven of *Death and Dying: The Tibetan Tradition* (London: Penguin Arkana, 1986).

22. Presumably this refers to his *Great Commentary to Transference* (Tib. '*Pho ba tik chen*).

23. There are many different accounts of Darma Dodey's death and the circumstances leading up to it. The most common is that Marpa had been instructed to give the sixth of Naropa's Six Yogas, that of forceful projection, exclusively to Milarepa, with the injunction that it must be kept extremely secret. Marpa instead gave it to his son Darma Dodey. This invoked the consternation of the yogic community, who feared that it would fall into the wrong hands. One of these yogis, Rva Lotsawa, known and feared in the spiritual community of eleventh-century Tibet as a self-appointed tantric policeman, visited Marpa and heavily chastised him for the transgression, informing him that the only solution was for him to put his own son to death. Marpa was unable to do so because of his paternal affection. Rva Lotsawa therefore performed a magical ritual, transformed himself into a crow, and knocked Darma Dodey off his horse and to his death.

24. Gyalwa Wensapa (b. 1505) is one of the great legends in Gelukpa mystical history and an early lineage holder of the Six Yogas transmission. He wrote quintessential guides to all the principal tantric systems preserved within the Gelukpa school. These dispense with the details in the practice and go directly to the underlying principles of the individual systems. His *A Source of Every Realization: The Stamp of the Six Yogas of Naropa* (Tib. *Na ro chos drug gi lag rjes dngos grub kun 'byung*) is typical of his literary style.

25. The most reliable account is to be found in Tsepon W. D. Shakabpa's *A Political History of Tibet* (New Haven: Yale University Press, 1967). This work is invaluable to an understanding of the dark side of Tibetan history.

In fact, Shakabpa probably gained his source materials from the notes of Gendun Chopel, the Amdo lama who had assisted George Roerich in the translation of *The Blue Annals*. Gendun Chopel was the first Tibetan lama to have exposure to the Western critical approach to historical analysis, and thus was capable of writing realistically on matters of conflict.

This is very different from traditional Tibetan biographical or historical writings, which either completely gloss over conflicts and problems, or else resort to a self-serving and self-righteous posture. Gendun Chopel, on the other hand, seems to have freely criticized anyone and everyone wherever he felt it appropriate.

Shakabpa was one of the officers who arrested Gendun Chopel for treason in 1950, after which Gendun Chopel's thousands of notes, gleaned from the Potala's vast archives, disappeared, never to be seen again. It seems too great a coincidence that Shakabpa later came out with a book having the quality and style of *A Political History of Tibet*. This was the opinion of young Tibetan intellectuals during my period of studies in India in the 1970s.

26. His Holiness the Dalai Lama once commented that if we were to examine the life of Tsongkhapa and calculate the amount of time he devoted to meditation, it would seem that he gave his entire life to contemplative practice. Similarly, if we were to look at the volume and depth of his writings, it would seem that he was always engaged in literary pursuits. And if we were to list the number of teachings he gave during his lifetime, it would seem that he was always teaching. "His most amazing quality," stated His Holiness, "was that he accomplished as much as ten ordinary people in all three spheres."

27. The practice of *chulen* (Tib. *bcud len*), or "taking the essence," is treated in *The Tantric Yogas of Sister Niguma* (Ithaca: Snow Lion Publications, 1984) in the Second Dalai Lama's text on making "essence pills" from flowers and then abstaining from any food and eating only a few of these pellets each day. While living in India I knew several yogis who thus cut off intake of ordinary food for two or three years at a time, eating only a pellet or two a day for sustenance. They lost weight for the first three or four months, but after that even became quite fat.

The three main forms of the practice are: pellets made from flower petals; pellets made from certain minerals; and "stone essence," in which a stone is put into a glass of water several times a day, mantras recited, and the water then drunk. The First Dalai Lama's writings mention a fourth technique: breathing in the essence of starlight at night. Starlight is considered to be the essence of energy, and thus the most quintessential form of nutrient.

A Book of Three Inspirations by Tsongkhapa the Great

1. Buddha Vajradhara is the tantric emanation of Shakyamuni, the historical buddha. He symbolizes the esoteric dimension of spiritual inspiration from which the highest yoga tantras were taught. He is the *Adibuddha*, or "Primordial Buddha," in all the New Schools of Tibetan Buddhism.

2. Chang utterly misconstrues this passage in his translation, mistaking the term *dung rab zinpa* (Tib. *gdung rabs 'dzin pa*), or "bone lineage holder," i.e., paternal blood line, for that of *la gyu zinpa* (Tib. *bla brgyud 'dzin pa*), or "guru lineage holder." The idea is that Miwang Drakpa Gyaltsen, the hereditary Pakmo Drupa ruler who requested Tsongkhapa the Great to clarify the tradition of Naro's Six Yogas by writing a commentary to it, was a great patron of yogis engaged in the intense practice of the Six Yogas. When Tsongkhapa says that this patron had achieved rebirth as "one holding the ancestral lineage /Of a being on the exalted platform of serving as chieftain / To fortunate trainees who applied themselves to this path...," Chang instead has him saying, "Following its path, the hard-working and gifted disciples / Are led to the plane of saviors." Tsongkhapa's meaning is not that these disciples are led to the path of saviors, but that Miwang Drakpa Gyaltsen was a great chieftain as well as being a great patron of practitioners.

Tibetans use the expression "bone lineage" for the paternal line, because their idea is that our skeletal structure evolves from our father's sperm, and our flesh and blood from our mother's ovum. This led to a unique sexual liberty for women; a Tibetan woman married to several brothers might take lovers from amongst her husband's immediate relatives, because the "bone lineage" of any offspring would remain the same. I have encountered several cases of this nature during my twenty years with Tibetans.

3. Here Tsongkhapa's shorter manual does not mention the general Mahayana preliminaries at all, and jumps directly into the "Vajrayana preliminaries that are exclusive to the Six Yogas tradition," i.e., the Vajrasattva and guru yoga meditations. Thus the discussion of the tantric initiations and Vajrayana *samaya* are also omitted. This is noteworthy in that, as we will see in the following section of his treatise, he speaks at such length on the importance of these preliminary trainings and conditions.

4. Tsongkhapa's wording, "Lama Ngokpa, who quotes *The Hevajra Tantra in Two Sections* as saying...," suggests that he is unsure of the passage yet nonetheless mentions it in order to show that Lama Ngokpa advocated using the general Mahayana teachings as a preliminary to the Six Yogas training.

Tsongkhapa gives only the first and last line of the verse, for he had obviously lifted it from Ngokpa's writings, where it appears in this form. I read through *The Hevajra Tantra in Two Sections* to find the passage and fill it out, but it is not to be found there. This would suggest either that Lama Ngokpa used a different edition of the text than the one eventually included in the Tibetan canon, or that he confused the source. I would guess the former situation to be the case, as every chapter of this tantra has a verse beginning with the line "firstly impart the precept...." Presumably Lama Tsongkhapa was aware that the passage was not to be found in the original tantra as presented in the Kangyur, and consequently he introduced it with words that link it to Ngokpa's writings, rather than directly to *The Hevajra Tantra in Two Sections* itself.

When the Tibetan canons were compiled and edited, standard forms of the translations of various Indian treatises were preserved. However, a negative side effect is that alternate translations, often made from different Indian editions, fell out of use and over the centuries were lost. It is possible that this occurred with the version of the *Hevajra Tantra* quoted by Lama Ngokpa.

5. Chang mistranslates this as "...the misfortune bringer always turns out to be one's best friend. The fallers in the abyss are the men who follow the cattle."

Tibet was a country of farmers and nomadic herdsmen. The image of one ox yoked to another in a plowing harness would have had a visceral impact on Tsongkhapa's readers. Throughout his translation Chang completely misses the raw earthiness and sheer drama of Tsongkhapa's style, which is characterized by a richness and a direct simplicity that caused him to become the single most popular writer in Central Asian history.

6. In other words, during Milarepa's time the expression *Bardo Drangdrol*, or "Achieving Liberation in the Bardo," was another name for the *Naro Choe Druk*, or "Naro's Six Dharmas." This probably derives from the threefold use of the term *bardo* in the Six Yogas system: the bardo between birth and death (i.e., waking-state life); the bardo of sleep and dreams; and the bardo that follows the moment of death.

7. "The Four Dharmas of Gampopa" refers both to a short text by Gampopa, and to a meditative tradition that the text inspired.

Ngulchu Dharmabhadra (b. 1722) explains in his *Ornament for A Book of Three Inspirations* (Tib. *Na ro chos drug gi zin bris yid ches dgongs rgyan*), "The four factors included in the tradition known as 'the Four Dharmas of Gampopa' are as follows: turning the mind to Dharma; turning Dharma into the path; using the path to eliminate confusion; and causing confusion to arise as primordial wisdom awareness."

8. Tsongkhapa wrote three separate treatises on the topic of the *Lam Rim*: extensive, intermediate and brief. The latter text, which is in verse, is also known as the *Lam Rim Nyamgur* (Tib. *Lam rim nyams mgur*), or *Song of the Lam Rim Experience*. This was used as the basis of the Third Dalai Lama's *Stages on the Path to Enlightenment: Essence of Refined Gold* (Tib. *Lam rim gser gyi yang zhun ma*), which I translated in my study of the Third Dalai Lama's life and teachings, *Selected Works of the Dalai Lama III: Essence of Refined Gold* (Ithaca: Snow Lion Publications, 1982). This has recently been reprinted under the title *The Path to Enlightenment* by the Dalai Lama (Ithaca: Snow Lion Publications, 1995). I would recommend it to any reader of the present text on Naropa's Six Yogas who would like to better understand the nature of the preliminaries to tantric practice. The Dalai Lama's contemporary elucidation of the Third Dalai Lama's classical treatise brings together the best of the modern and ancient Tibetan worlds.

9. Atisha Dipamkara Shrijnana, the Indian master who came to Tibet in 1042, is regarded not only as the forefather of the Kadampa school, but as an important influence on all the New Schools—Kargyu, Sakya and Geluk. Gampopa's *Lam Rim Tar Gyan* (Tib. *Lam rim thar rgyan*), or *Jewel Ornament of Liberation* (translated by Herbert Guenther; London, 1959), is popularly known to Tibetans as "The Union of Two Streams," the two being Milarepa's lineages and those of Atisha.

Tsongkhapa's reference here to Atisha is relevant to his purposes for two reasons. Firstly, the *Lam Rim* legacy mentioned earlier in *A Book of Three Inspirations* has its root in Atisha's *A Lamp for the Path to Enlightenment* (Skt. *Bodhipathapradipa*), a contemplative tradition that was wholeheartedly incorporated by Tsongkhapa. In fact, his three *Lam Rim* treatises are largely inspired by it. Secondly, this same *Lam Rim* tradition from Atisha was incorporated by Gampopa and fused with the lineages he received from Milarepa, including that of the Six Yogas of Naropa. Thus Atisha's lineage became an important basis for both the Geluk and Kargyu schools.

10. The wording of Tsongkhapa's text here is intended to link these preliminaries to the teaching popular in the Kargyu schools under the name *lodok namzhi* (Tib. *blo ldok rnam bzhi*), or "Four Ways of Turning the Mind," which refers to the general Mahayana meditations that are cultivated in order to prepare the mind for tantric practice. Tsongkhapa uses this Kargyu terminology because the Six Yogas of Naropa, the subject of his commentary, is a Kargyu lineage.

11. *Fifty Verses on the Guru*: This is a short text in fifty verses, penned by the Indian master and poet Ashvaghosha, that is held in great regard by Tibetans. It serves as the basic guideline to how the disciple should view and behave around the tantric guru. An English translation of it, rendered by Sharpa Tulku and Alex Berzin, is available from the Library of Tibetan Works and Archives, Dharamsala, India.

The Thirteenth Dalai Lama comments on the importance and nature of this brief text in "A Guide to the Buddhist Tantras," which is translated in my *Path of the Bodhisattva Warrior* (Ithaca: Snow Lion Publications, 1988):

> In the Resultant Vajrayana, even more so than in the Causal Sutrayana, it is said to be extremely important to train under the guidance of a qualified tantric master, to avoid wrong attitudes toward him and to cultivate positive attitudes, and to remain within the framework of the vows and commitments of the tantric path. In order to be able to do this it is useful to know the beneficial effects of conducive attitudes and the shortcomings of faulty attitudes, how to regard the guru's entourage and possessions, the nature of correct and incorrect practice, and so forth. All these topics are discussed in detail in *The Root Tantra of Guhyasamaja* (Skt. *Guhyasamaja mula tantra*), the *Hevajra Tantra in Two Sections* (Skt. *Hevajra tantra nama*), ...and other texts. The general themes on how to rely correctly upon the vajra guru were gleaned from these early source works and collected into fifty quintessential verses, entitled *Fifty Verses on the Guru* (Skt. *Guru panchashika karika*) by Acharya Vira, who was also known by the names Aryashura and Ashvaghosha.

12. This probably refers to his three *Lam Rim* treatises, mentioned in note 8 above.

13. Chang mistranslates this passage as, "When Milarepa first saw Gambopa [sic], he asked Gambopa whether he had obtained the complete initiations before imparting the teachings of the Six Yogas. Gambopa replied, 'Like a copper

utensil ready for filling with butter, I am quite ready.' Thereupon, Milarepa be-
stowed upon him the teachings and Pith Instructions."

Here Chang seems to have totally misread the name of one of Gampopa's
early initiation gurus, Maryul Loden (Tib. Mar yul blo ldan), and also this master's
guru, Zangkar Lotsawa (Tib. Zangs dkar). *Mar* means "red," and *yul* means
"land"; the two together refer to a district in Western Tibet. *Loden* (Tib. blo ldan)
is a common Buddhist name meaning wise or wisdom. Thus his name was Red
Land Sage. Zangkar is the name of a province of Ladakh, and also of a famous
early eleventh-century translator from that region. Here it refers to the lama.
Chang seems to have taken *Mar* to mean "butter," and the first syllable of *Zangkar*
to mean "copper." This forced him into his erroneous reading.

He also gets the next line backwards: "On another occasion, before Milarepa
gave Gampopa an oral transmission teaching, he sent him to receive empowerments from Bari Lotsawa." Chang has this as, "Milarepa also urged Gambopa to
encourage the Bari Translator to come for initiations." It is not the Buddhist tradition for gurus to beg others to come to their teachings or initiations.

14. These are the first two of the six phases of the "vase" empowerment. The
vase empowerment in turn is the first of the four empowerments given to aspir-
ants wishing to enter into highest yoga tantra practice. It is called "vase empowerment" because each of its phases concludes with the sprinkling of sacred waters from the initiation vase. The first five of these six steps introduces the disciple to the five Tathagata families, transforming the five distorted emotions
into the five wisdoms and the five psychophysical aggregates into the five
Tathagatas, thus authorizing the trainee to take up the generation stage yogas
and also planting the seeds of the Nirmanakaya. The sixth vase empowerment
is that of the vajra master, authorizing the trainee to later give empowerment to
others after the completion of his or her training.

The concluding three empowerments are called secret, wisdom awareness
and sacred word.

15. The blessing initiation, or *jenang* (Tib. *rje nang*; lit., subsequent transmission)
is a simpler form of empowerment and should only be given to those who have
previously received a complete empowerment into the class of mandala being
imparted. The "blessing initiation" does not have the standard stages of initiation, such as vase and so forth, but only has a blessing or communion of "body,
speech and mind" of the mandala deity.

These days the understanding of the distinction seems to be hazy, and lamas
quite randomly give a public *jenang* without ensuring that participants have
previously received the qualifying empowerments. To do so is said to degener-
ate the tantric tradition, and to be harmful to both the initiating master and the
recipient.

His Holiness the Dalai Lama once pointed this out in an audience I had with
him, and then laughed, adding, "I suspect that even highly educated lamas do
this on their Western tours, with thoughts of getting a larger offering from the
larger crowds."

16. Here Ngulchu Dharmabhadra states in his *Ornament for A Book of Three Inspirations* (Tib. *Na ro chos drug gi zin bris yid ches dgongs rgyan*),

> The meaning of 'the four complete initiations' [in Tsongkhapa's text] is that one should receive the four complete initiations into the appropriate highest yoga tantra system, such as any of the three Heruka Chakrasamvara lineages—those of Luipada, Krishnacharya or Ghantapada—or any of the four types of Hevajra—the Oral Transmission Lineage, the Dombipa Lineage, the Padma Lineage, or the Krishnacharya Lineage.

17. Jey Sherab Gyatso (b. 1803) states in *Notes on A Book of Three Inspirations* (Tib. *Yid ches gsum ldan gyi shad lung zin bris*),

> The discussion of the manner of maintaining the samaya and guidelines are discussed in detail in the four texts famed as 'The Four Great Treatises on the Preliminary Practices' (Tib. *sNgon 'gro khrid chen bzhi*), which are popular in other schools such as the Sakya, Nyingma, and so forth. Although there is nothing directly from the hand of Tsongkhapa the Great that deals with the preliminaries in that manner, i.e., with both the general Sutrayana and exclusive Vajrayana preliminaries in one text, he has written extensively on the Sutrayana trainings [in his *Lam Rim* treatises], and referred to the Vajrayana preliminaries in various of his tantric works....

18. Here Jey Sherab Gyatso mentions in his *Notes on A Book of Three Inspirations* that the Vajrasattva meditation exhibits a predominance of the color white. This is because each of the four types of tantric activity—pacification, amplification, empowerment and destruction—is associated with its own color: white, yellow, red and dark blue, respectively, and in the Vajrasattva practice the emphasis is on the first of these, or pacification. The object of this pacification is negative karma and obscuration; these are purified by means of the meditation and mantra recitation. Hence Vajrasattva is white in color, as are the five buddhas who come into the space above the meditator and pour forth purifying nectars. The nectars that they pour are also white in color. Similarly, if a more complex Vajrasattva mandala with four consorts is used, all of these are white.

Jey Sherab Gyatso also comments that with the guru yoga meditation it is important that one imagine one's body, speech and mind to be inseparable in nature from the body, speech and mind of the guru (who is visualized as Buddha Vajradhara), and that this point of communion of the three be seen as arising in the nature of the three kayas of the yidam, or mandala deity. Similarly, one's own suchness nature is seen as being inseparable from the suchness nature of the guru, and this arises as the yidam. Sherab Gyatso comments, "This dynamic brings about rapid attainment of siddhi."

19. The first three of Marpa Lotsawa's four chief disciples—Mey (Tib. Mes), Tsur (Tib. 'Tshur), Ngok (Tib. rNgogs) and Milarepa (Tib. Mi la ras pa) are referred to in various ways throughout Tsongkhapa's manual. Mey occasionally becomes Lama Mey, and also Meyton. Tsur is alternately Lama Tsur and Tsurton. Ngok

appears as Lama Ngok, Lama Ngokpa, Ngokpa and also Ngokton. Here the syllable *ton* (Tib. *ston*) that is sometimes suffixed to their names means "teacher" or "spiritual master." Goe Lotsawa provides brief biographies of all four in *The Blue Annals*.

20. In other words, the lamas of the Six Yogas tradition who teach that the generation stage yogas are unnecessary contradict the instructions of their own lineage masters. Tsongkhapa quotes the verse from Milarepa to prove his point.

21. Ngulchu Dharmabhadra explains the etymology of the term "generation stage yoga" as follows in *An Ornament for A Book of Three Inspirations:* "It is called 'generation stage yoga' because one meditates by generating the vision [of the mandala and its deities] as symbolic of the process of life, death and bardo."

He continues,

> All of Marpa's four chief disciples were first led through the generation stage practice before being led through the completion stage. The reason is that the generation stage process ripens and prepares the mind of the trainee for the realizations that are brought to fulfillment by means of the completion stage yogas. Moreover, the deity yoga meditations practiced during the generation stage introduce the subject of ordinary birth, death and bardo, and point the mind to how these three occasions are transformed into a path to enlightenment, until eventually the three are brought into the state of the resultant three kayas of full enlightenment.

22. Ngulchu Dharmabhadra gives the list of these four "families of Hevajra" in *An Ornament for A Book of Three Inspirations* (see note 16 above). Ngulchu uses the term *rig* (Tib. *rigs*), or "family," rather than *luk* (Tib. *lugs*), or "lineage," but his list clearly identifies them as individual transmissions.

23. Here Tsongkhapa mentions three different transmissions of the Indian mahasiddha Luipa's lineage of Heruka Chakrasamvara.

The first of them is the Zangkar lineage. We saw a reference to this earlier in the discussion of what empowerments are appropriate as the basis of practicing the Six Yogas of Naropa. Gampopa received this from Maryul Loden, a disciple of Zangkar the Translator. As I pointed out in note 13 above, Chang mistakes the name of Maryul Loden, translating it as "butter," and takes the name of Maryul Loden's lama, i.e., Lama Zangkar, to mean "copper vessel." When Tsongkhapa says, "Gampopa relied upon the lineage of Maryul Loden, the disciple of Zangkar (Lotsawa)... known as 'the Chakrasamvara lineage of Zangkar...,'" Chang has him saying, "From Gamboba, through the transmission of Ladak and Mar, the Bde mchog teaching of Ladak was transmitted."

He also mistakes the second lineage, in which Tsongkhapa says, "Also, the glorious Pakmo Drupa relied upon the Chakrasamvara transmission from Lochung, known as the Mar Lineage." Chang has him saying, "In his youth the Glorious Pag-mo-grub-pa practiced the Bde-mchog from Mar-do." Here *Lochung* does not mean "...in his youth"; rather, it is the popular name of a famous translator from Western Tibet known as Lochung, or "The Junior Translator."

In the third passage Tsongkhapa says, "Moreover, the Dharma master Chojey Drikungpa relied upon the Chakrasamvara tradition of Lama Chokro, which is the lineage from Mardo (Tib. Mar do)." Chang omits this important lineage altogether, and shuffles it into what was being said earlier about Pakmo Drupa's lineage.

Concerning the second of the three lineages mentioned above, Lochung was one of the two especially great translators who appeared in Western Tibet during the eleventh century. These two are popularly known to Tibetan history as Lochen and Lochung, or "Senior Translator" and "Junior Translator." These could also be rendered as "the Elder" and "the Younger," or as "the Greater" and "the Lesser." All that is meant is that one predates the other.

The former is none other than the illustrious Lochen Rinchen Zangpo, who inspired the renaissance of the eleventh century, and was said to be eighty years of age when Atisha arrived in Tibet in 1042. He became a disciple of Atisha, and after meeting him went into solitary retreat for the duration of his life. His endorsement of Atisha undoubtedly contributed greatly to the respect that Atisha was thereafter shown in Tibet, for at the time Lochen Rinchen Zangpo was considered the greatest spiritual master in the country. His *tulku*, or official reincarnation, lives in India today.

Lochung, or "Junior Translator," was a disciple of Lochen Rinchen Zangpo, and also became a disciple of Atisha. According to *The Blue Annals*, this is none other than Ngok Lekpai Sherab. I tell something of his life in *Verses of a Mad Dalai Lama* (Wheaton, IL: Quest Books, 1994).

24. Chang again here totally misreads the passage and confuses the various Chakrasamvara mandalas that Tsongkhapa is recommending. This passage is discussed above in the introduction.

Jey Sherab Gyatso comments in his *Notes on A Book of Three Inspirations*, "Marpa Lotsawa himself used both the Hevajra and Heruka Chakrasamvara mandalas." What he means is that Marpa would teach either as the basis of the Six Yogas.

25. The coarse and subtle generation stage yogas: The former refers to visualizing the supporting and supported mandalas; the latter refers to doing this while simultaneously envisioning the entire mandala as being inside a drop the size of a sesame seed. The difference is in the degree of meditative concentration that has been attained.

26. Ngulchu Dharmabhadra's *An Ornament for A Book of Three Inspirations* states,

> If one appreciates the nature of the basis [i.e., the deeper nature of the body and mind], one will come to know the nature of the path. And through understanding the nature of the path one engages in spiritual practice and comes to actualize the nature of the result, which is enlightenment.

27. Ngulchu Dharmabhadra comments in *An Ornament for A Book of Three Inspirations*,

> The approach to emptiness meditation in the tradition of the Six Yogas of Naropa is slightly unlike the approaches found in other highest

yoga tantra systems of completion stage practice. Here the emphasis is upon ascertaining the ultimate nature of being by means of the meditational process in its causal context.

What he means by this is that in other completion stage systems the emphasis in the technique is upon resting within a proxy of the primordial wisdom and the resultant enlightenment mind, whereas in the Six Yogas system the emphasis is upon meditation on emptiness as a causal means of arousing that primordial wisdom.

28. When Tsongkhapa points out the necessity of integrating the vision of emptiness into conventional daily life, Chang utterly mistakes what is being said and comments in note 55, "Here is shown Tsong Khapa's timidness on Sunyata, and his materialistic view is clearly reflected." The reason why the Indian schools descending from Nagarjuna and Aryadeva call themselves the Madhyamaka, or "Middle View"—and all Tibetan sects claim to be based on the Indian Madhyamaka schools—is that they avoid the two extremes of reification and nihilism. This is expressed in classical Madhyamaka treatises by saying that the syndrome of reification is eliminated through appreciating how all things are empty of true existence; and the syndrome of nihilism is eliminated by appreciating how all things simultaneously function with validity on the conventional level according to the infallible laws of interdependence and causality. As for a "timidness" toward emptiness, Tsongkhapa wrote half a dozen treatises on the topic, several of which are hundreds of pages in length. Even a casual glance at what he has to say will dispel any concept that he was shy of the subject, or that his view was materialistic.

29. Tsongkhapa's presentation of the nature of the body here is rather sparse, and leaves out the discussion of the three or four physical dimensions or "sheathes." The commentary by Gyalwa Wensapa, *A Source of Every Realization: The Stamp of the Six Yogas of Naropa* (Tib. *Na ro chos drug gi lag rjes dngos grub kun 'byung*) gives a wonderful presentation of this fundamental aspect of tantric theory. See the "Introduction to the Nature of the Body" section of the introduction.

30. Ngulchu Dharmabhadra comments in his *An Ornament for A Book of Three Inspirations*,

> The physical exercises and the meditations upon the body as an empty shell are not described in any of the authentic Indian tantric scriptures. It seems that they are based exclusively on the oral tradition of the gurus. When they are performed, there is less chance of problematic side effects arising in the channels or energies through forceful meditation on the tantric yogas; and even if some difficulties do arise, these are mitigated.

At his 1991 discourse His Holiness commented that he thought perhaps these two techniques were developed by the early Tibetan masters.

31. Ngulchu Dharmabhadra's treatment of these various arrangements is discussed in the introduction, in the "Legacy of the Six Yogas" section.

Nagtsang Tulku, a lama who attained to prominence in the late nineteenth century, wrote a wonderful practice manual on the Six Yogas system, entitled *A Source of Great Bliss Realization: A Guide to the Profound Six Yogas of Naropa*, in which he uses an approach quite different from that of Tsongkhapa. He divides the completion stage practices of the Six Yogas system into two: meditating on the inner heat and thus giving rise to the four blisses; and, secondly, on the basis of that realization, the meditations on "the (nine) blendings."

In his treatment of the inner heat yoga he by-passes the elaborate system of outlines followed by Tsongkhapa and instead presents it in eight simple steps in practice: (1) the breathing exercises for expelling dead energies/air, together with the physical exercises; (2) visualizing the energy channels; (3) purifying the pathways of the channels; (4) visualizing the mantric syllables in the chakras; (5) kindling the fire of the inner heat; (6) causing the fire of the inner heat to blaze; (7) how the practitioner brings about blazing and melting/falling of the mystic drops; and (8) the special applications of blazing and melting/falling.

We can see that here, unlike Tsongkhapa, he presents the physical exercises and meditations on the body as an empty shell as the first step in the inner heat training, and not as a preliminary.

32. Marpa taught the Six Yogas differently to different disciples. Milarepa received only the "oral instruction transmission" (Tib. *man ngag gi brgyud*). Lama Ngok and Lama Tsur received the teaching complete with all the source tantras and tantric shastras; thus their lineages are known as "explanatory lineages" (Tib. *bshad brgyud*).

33. "Secret whispered tradition" (Tib. *snyan brgyud*) refers to an oral instruction transmission that is always transmitted orally. Marpa used the term as a synonym for his tantric teachings.

34. The four exalted transmissions of Naropa: The Nalanda Translation Committee point out in a footnote to their translation *The Life of Marpa the Translator* (Boulder: Prajna, 1982, pp. xxxii-xxxiii) that there are various ways of describing these four. They are most frequently seen as "the four instructions of Tilopa," for they were first given by Tilopa to Naropa, and then later imparted by Naropa to Marpa. The tradition of the Six Yogas of Naropa derives from them. *The Life of Marpa the Translator* provides three different versions of these four.

Ngulchu Dharmabhadra gives them as inner heat, karmamudra, illusory body, and clear light. See also "The Legacy of the Six Yogas" in the introduction.

35. A wonderful account of the transmissions discussed here by Tsongkhapa can be found in greater detail in Taranatha's *The Seven Instruction Lineages* (Tib. *bKa' babs bdun ldan*), translated by David Templeman (Dharamsala: Library of Tibetan Works and Archives, 1983). The Tibetan historian Taranatha (b. 1575) provides the names of the gurus in seven principal tantric lineages, as well as summaries of their biographies. The names of most of the Indian mahasiddhas quoted by Tsongkhapa in *A Book of Three Inspirations* can be found in Taranatha's text. These seven lineages contribute important elements of the Six Yogas of Naropa, and thus Templeman's book is highly recommended to anyone wanting further historical background on the Naropa system.

36. Tibetans generally use an abbreviation of the Sanskrit name of the central channel, reducing *avadhuti* to *dhuti*. They sometimes also call it *tsa uma* (Tib. *rtsa dbu ma*). For the two side channels, *rasana* and *lalana*, they use *roma* (Tib. *rtsa ro ma*) and *kyangma* (Tib. *rtsa brkyang ma*), respectively.

37. Ngulchu Dharmabhadra explains the "lotus petals" of the energy channels as follows in *An Ornament for A Book of Three Inspirations*:

> At the navel chakra an energy channel petal reaches into each of the four directions; these four then split into two, making eight; these split into two, making sixteen; these split into two, making thirty-two; and finally these also split into two each, making sixty-four.

He goes on to explain how the eight at the heart chakra, sixteen at the throat chakra, thirty-two at the crown chakra and sixty-four at the navel chakra are formed in the same manner, beginning with four that branch out to eight, and so forth.

He also points out that the channel petals at the navel flow upward, like an overturned umbrella, and those at the heart flow downward, like an upright umbrella. The same is the case with the "petals" of the chakras at the throat and crown. This is what Tsongkhapa means here when he says, "...within an according embrace of method and wisdom."

38. Lawapa (Skt. Lvavapada) also plays an important role in the transmission of this doctrine, and thus is mentioned several times throughout Tsongkhapa's treatise. He was the guru of Jalandaripa, who in turn was the guru of Krishnacharya, mentioned below. His story is told by Taranatha in *The Seven Instruction Lineages*.

39. Tsongkhapa refers to Krishnacharya several times in this section of *A Book of Three Inspirations*, because this Indian master plays an important role in the transmission of both the Hevajra and Chakrasamvara tantric cycles. These are the two principal tantric sources of the inner heat doctrine as received by Tilopa and transmitted to Naropa. The Tibetan historian Taranatha is an excellent source for knowledge of his life and works. See David Templeman's translation, *Taranatha's Life of Krishnacarya/Kanha* (Dharamsala: Library of Tibetan Works and Archives, 1989).

40. *Padmini* (Tib. Pad ma can) is both the name of a well-known tenth-century Indian female tantrika and the title of a tantric treatise in the Heruka Chakrasamvara cycle.

41. I did not have access to the collected works of Pakmo Drupa during the period of my writing, and thus was unable to check these two compositions, his verse and prose writings on the Six Doctrines. Tsongkhapa refers to both throughout this treatise.

42. Ngulchu Dharmabhadra states in *An Ornament for A Book of Three Inspirations* that this vase breathing technique also has great health benefits and is widely used in the tantric yogas for self-healing. I personally have seen it taught in this context, as illustrated by a work by the First Dalai Lama (b. 1391) on the eight

generation stage and eight completion stage yogas of the Amitayus/Hayagriva tantric cycle having its origins in the Nepalese female mystic Siddharani.

43. The mantric *AH*-stroke at the navel is sometimes referred to as *AM* (or the *AM*-stroke) in Tsongkhapa's text, presumably because of the crescent of half moon, sun and *nada* above it, The sun symbol in the crescent is also used in the Tibetan script to denote the sound of the suffix letter "M." Thus the syllable *AH* with a crescent can also signify the sound of *AM*. The manner of visualization of the two, *AH* and *AM*, would remain the same, i.e., a perpendicular stroke with its crescent.

44. His Holiness the Dalai Lama laughed when explaining this traditional manner of counting, and said that many yogis would lose the number of the count in the attempt to test themselves. Consequently the system of counting has been replaced by a simpler method. With the fingers of the right hand one taps the right knee, left knee and forehead, and then slowly snaps the fingers three times in front of the heart. The number of times one repeats this cycle is counted, and one's competence in the practice is measured as best, intermediate or least, based on whether the cycle is 108, 72 or 36.

45. There is a considerable amount of literature in English on sexual yoga as practiced in the Hindu tantric traditions of India, and also as practiced in the Taoist traditions of China. The Buddhist tantrikas have over the centuries emphasized secrecy with this aspect of tantric training, and have restricted their knowledge of the sexual meditative techniques to initiates.

46. At this point in his commentary Nagtsang Tulku's *A Source of Great Bliss Realization: A Guide to the Profound Six Yogas of Naropa* explains the process of arising with the illusory body in the language of the "nine blendings," as discussed in the introduction.

Perhaps the best English-language account of the principles of illusory body and clear light as taught in the Guhyasamaja Tantra, the source of these doctrines in the Six Yogas system, is Daniel Cozort's *Highest Yoga Tantra* (Ithaca: Snow Lion Publications, 1986). Cozort's discussion of the doctrine of final mind refinement and its relation to the illusory body doctrine, pages 89-95, are relevant to what Tsongkhapa is saying here.

47. Here Ngulchu Dharmabhadra makes the rather interesting comment, "The place at which this illusory body is produced for the first time is within one's old aggregates, at the center of the heart chakra." He also states, "The meditational technology for both the illusory body and clear light doctrines in the Six Yogas system comes from the Guhyasamaja Tantra, and is based upon the Arya Cycle of Guhyasamaja as transmitted by Marpa Lotsawa himself."

A Book of Three Inspirations presents the Guhyasamaja ideas in a few pages; anyone wanting a more elaborate picture is referred to Daniel Cozort's *Highest Yoga Tantra*.

48. As Lama Tsongkhapa implies in this treatise, and as Jey Sherab Gyatso points out more explicitly in *Notes on A Book of Three Inspirations*, these three levels of

training in the illusory nature of experience are really intended for beginners. Jey Sherab Gyatso states,

> The early Tibetan masters, such as Marpa, Milarepa and so forth, primarily taught these methods in order to plant instincts on the mindstream of practitioners on initial stages in the training.... The actual illusory body yoga...is practiced in the house assembled at the center of the heart chakra from the substance of the white and red drops.

49. Here Tsongkhapa is simply pointing out that one must appreciate the ultimate level of reality, the emptiness nature of all existents, in light of the conventional reality of how things function with validity on the ordinary level. That is to say, even though all things ultimately are void of a self nature, on the conventional level there are living beings who hear sounds, see things, engage in activities, create karma through their actions and then experience the according results, and so forth.

Chang writes in his footnote 82, "This statement reflects Tsong Khapa's philosophy of Voidness to the effect that all conceptions are Void (Empty), but that beings themselves exist."

In fact Tsongkhapa is not saying this at all, and clearly regards living beings as every bit as void of self-nature as inanimate phenomena. He follows in the footsteps of the classical Indian Madhyamaka masters Nagarjuna, Aryadeva and Chandrakirti, and thus teaches that all existents ultimately lack true existence, yet nonetheless on the conventional level of reality continue to function with validity. "Conceptions" and "living beings" are no different in this respect. Thoughts, living beings, buddhas, worms, tables and elephants all equally abide in the one-tasteness of emptiness as their ultimate nature; yet conventionally, based on names, labels and mental imputation, they function according to the laws of cause and effect. Nagarjuna dedicates Chapter 24 of his most famous and quintessential work, *Verses on the Middle View* (Skt. *Madhyamaka karika shastra*), to this very point.

50. Ngulchu Dharmabhadra's *Ornament for A Book of Three Inspirations* presents the doctrine of "the bardo of becoming," i.e., the bardo that is experienced between death and rebirth, together with the nature of the bardo body, under thirteen topics. These are as follows: (1) etymology: it is called "the bardo of becoming" because it comes into being from the mind's inner visions; (2) physical nature: it is born from mind and the subtle energy seeds carried by the mind, and appears with all senses complete; (3) form: one assumes the form of the world into which one will take rebirth; (4) color: when good karma is the driving force, one's body is the color of white moonlight; when driven by negative karma it is the color of dark clouds at night; (5) seeming age: when orienting toward rebirth in the world of sensuality, or the *kamadhatu*, it appears as between five and ten years of age; (6) sense of motion: when propelled toward a lower rebirth there is the sensation of descending; when propelled toward rebirth as a ghost or animal there is a sense of wandering on a flatland; and when a high rebirth as a human, asura or deva is indicated, the sense is of moving upward; (7) abilities of

cognizance: it perceives companions of a form similar to itself, and has the five clairvoyances; (8) sustenance: it consumes only scents and aromas; (9) behavioral patterns: it is propelled by the positive and negative karmic instincts that it carries within itself; (10) powers and strengths: it can instantly and miraculously travel anywhere in the universe without obstruction, with the exception of its future place of rebirth; (11) signs: there is no sun or moon in the sky, the body casts no shadow and leaves no footprints, those to whom one calls out do not seem to hear and do not reply, and there are fearful sounds, such as of windstorms, earthquakes, etc.; (12) duration: its life span is indefinite, but lasts a maximum of seven times seven cycles; and (13) its manner of taking rebirth: if by miraculous birth, there is an attraction to the place of rebirth; if the birth mode is by heat/metamorphosis, the attraction is to the aroma of the place; and if the birth is to be by egg or womb, the bardo being sees the copulating parents to be, and develops attraction for the parent of the sex opposite to that it will take, and aversion for the parent of the same sex.

51. These two fourth-century Indian scriptures, the *Abhidharma kosha* by Vasubandhu and the *Abhidharma samucchaya* by his brother Asanga, are both very popular with Tibetans. The former is the more widely studied, and is part of the curriculum of all large Gelukpa monastic universities. Many of the Tibetan attitudes toward the nature of the afterlife derive from it.

52. When the term "bardo" is used in this threefold way, it encompasses the totality of sentient experience. During Milarepa's lifetime (b. 1040) the Six Yogas tradition was therefore known by the name *Bardo Trangdol gyi Menngak*, "The Oral Transmission for Achieving Liberation in the Bardo." Tsongkhapa mentions this in the preliminary sections of *A Book of Three Inspirations*, and it is discussed in the "Six Yogas, Three Bardo States, and Nine Blendings" section of the introduction.

As Tsongkhapa explains, because the Six Yogas system speaks of three bardo states, it must also speak of three illusory bodies, i.e., one for each of the three bardos. Thus there is the illusory body produced in meditation during the waking state; the illusory body experienced in dreams; and the illusory body that is the bardo form.

53. This important text by the Indian master Aryadeva is referred to several times by Tsongkhapa in *A Book of Three Inspirations*. It is a commentary to Nagarjuna's *Five Stages* (Skt. *Pancha krama*). Because Aryadeva was Nagarjuna's chief disciple and Dharma heir, this work is considered to be the most authoritative Indian guide to Nagarjuna's important breakdown of the Guhyasamaja tantric system. As stated earlier, the illusory body and clear light doctrines in the Six Yogas of Naropa are derived from the Guhyasamaja system, so Aryadeva's commentary is especially relevant here.

54. Again, Ngulchu Dharmabhadra clarifies the practice in his *An Ornament for A Book of Three Inspirations*:

> The special application of the consciousness transference practice is as follows. As before, one meditates on the inner heat practice and the vase breathing technique in order to draw the energies into the

central channel. This is said to be integral to the process. One should also engage in the six physical exercises as taught earlier, and perform the meditation on the body as an empty shell for a few moments. The three channels are visualized as before, with emphasis on the clarity of the central channel. In the gateway of the upper aperture stands a white syllable *KSHA*, its head pointing downward [i.e., standing upside down], thus blocking the channel. Again, the chakras at the heart and navel are visualized as before.

The two side channels join the central channel at the site of the lower aperture, four finger-widths below the navel. One meditates as before on the *AH*-stroke syllable that stands on a moon disc at the navel chakra. Also, one envisions the heart chakra, its petals pointing downward, like an inverted half moon... the long *HUM* syllable standing on a moon disc upon it, its head pointing downward, seat of the life-sustaining energies... one's mind, like an image reflected in a mirror, between the *U* vowel and the *HA* portion of the *HUM*.

55. As Ngulchu points out, the process described in the previous note causes the energies to be drawn into the central channel, rise, and strike the *AH* stroke, thus igniting the mystic fire. The energies then rise to the *HUM* at the heart chakra and strike the life-supporting energies there, causing the *HUM* to reverse its position and stand upright. The life energies, together with the syllable *HUM*, then rise to the *KSHA* at the crown. This then descends to the heart, where again the *HUM* takes its place, standing with head downward. This process is repeated again and again, and is practiced in four daily sessions.

56. Ngulchu's *An Ornament for A Book of Three Inspirations* gives these eight as follows: mouth, navel, sexual organ, anus, "treasury," nose, eyes and ears. He adds that the "Great Commentary" to the Six Yogas system written by Yongdzin Pandita, a text said to be the most extensive Gelukpa treatise on the Six Yogas of Naropa, states that the practitioner on more initial levels can simply concentrate on the central channel to effect the transference, without blocking these eight with mantric syllables. The term "treasury" above probably refers to the forehead aperture.

All eight of these apertures are to be "blocked by mantric syllables," as Tsongkhapa describes in the passages that follow.

57. Concerning the tantric assistant, Ngulchu's *Ornament for A Book of Three Inspirations* just adds, "He or she should be well embellished with the tantric samaya, and skilled in tantric activities."

58. Daniel Cozort translates these as "elaborative," "non-elaborative," and "very non-elaborative." See Daniel Cozort, *Highest Yoga Tantra* (Snow Lion Publications, 1986), pp. 91-93. However, Tsongkhapa gives the three a slightly different definition than does the nineteenth-century lama Ngawang Palden, the author of the Tibetan text upon which Cozort's book is based.

Ngulchu Dharmabhadra states in *An Ornament for A Book of Three Inspirations*,

In general, activities are of three levels. For those with inclinations for the lesser way there are the activities that avoid desire and sexuality. For those with inclinations for the vast ways there are the activities of creative deeds and the paramitas. Finally, for those with inclinations toward the profound path there are the activities that utilize desire and sexual energy.

In other words, "activities" can be considered within the context of any of the three yanas—Hinayana, Mahayana and Vajrayana.

Ngulchu continues,

> As for the third of these, they are of three types, known as "with embellishment," "without embellishment," and "utterly without embellishment." These three apply to both the generation and completion stage levels of practice.

59. Ngulchu Dharmabhadra again clarifies Tsongkhapa's meaning in *An Ornament for A Book of Three Inspirations*:

> The special activities are used by those proficient in the coarse and subtle generation stage in order to bypass the need to engage in the tantric ritual activities such as pacification, increase, power and wrath, and instead go directly to the eight magical powers. For someone who has already attained meditative stabilization, these eight are accomplished in as quick a time as seven days when they rely upon these special activities.
>
> As for the activities termed "with embellishment" and "without embellishment," in both cases they refer to engaging in the practice from within the sphere of awareness of the suchness nature of being. In general, one indulges in the sensual activities as the path, and in particular indulges in sex yoga with a karmamudra. In the former case [i.e., activities with embellishment] the yogi and yogini engage in the activity together with such embellishments as wearing erotic clothing, singing, dancing, and so forth. In the later case the yogi and yogini engage in the activities with minimal embellishment.
>
> Finally, "activities utterly without embellishment" refers to not engaging in practice with an actual sexual partner, or karmamudra, but instead doing so with a jnanamudra, or visualized dakini.

60. Jey Sherab Gyatso states in *Notes on A Book of Three Inspirations* (Tib. *Yid ches gsum ldan gyi shad lung zin bris*),

> There is also a "Treasure Text" source of the Six Yogas, but Tsongkhapa writes that he has no confidence in it whatsoever. This is the only occasion in Lama Tsongkhapa's writings in which he directly criticizes the Treasure Text tradition; at least, I am not aware of him doing so elsewhere.

The Tibetan text says *ter ney ton* (Tib. *gter nas bton*), or "revealed as treasures." This refers to a genre of literature in the Nyingma (Old Schools of Tibetan Buddhism) and Bonpo (pre-Buddhist) that emerged after the civil wars of the seventh and eighth centuries, in which most of Tibet's libraries were destroyed. Historically the first texts of this nature were *bey ter* (Tib. *sbas gter*), or "buried treasures," because in an attempt to save their literature both sides hid their books from wandering armies by burying them or hiding them in caves. Many of the people who had done so died before the texts were taken out, and as a result these were only discovered in future decades or centuries, if at all. Nyingma writers stated (and all later Buddhist historians have reiterated) that the Bonpos had no literature; but this is strongly contested by Western scholars such as David Snellgrove and contemporary Tibetan scholars such as Namkhai Norbu.

In later centuries there arose the popular belief in "buried treasures" that purportedly had been composed and hidden by Guru Padmasambhava, the Indian tantric master who had visited Tibet in the mid-eighth century. According to popular belief, Padmasambhava had written and concealed hundreds of these scriptures, with the thought that they would be revealed in and by future generations when the appropriate time had come.

Later on the traditions of "dream treasures" (Tib. *mi lam gter ma*), "meditation treasures" (Tib. *dgongs gter*), and "visionary revelations" (Tib. *dag snang*) emerged. Some of Tibet's greatest literature can be found in these three genres. Unlike buried treasures, which are rather simplistic in style, these three later forms of Nyingmapa and Bonpo literature are born from wonderful spiritual inspiration.

61. Concerning these two personages who had requested Tsongkhapa the Great to compose his treatise, Jey Sherab Gyatso's *Notes on A Book of Three Inspirations* (Tib. *Yid ches gsum ldan gyi shad lung zin bris*) states,

> Tsongkhapa's text was composed at the request of two brothers from the Pakmo Drupa family: Miwang Drakpa Gyaltsen, who was the principal sponsor of the Great Prayer Festival [which Tsongkhapa founded in 1409], and his younger brother Chojey Sonam Gyaltsen.

The elder brother, in accordance with Tibetan medieval tradition, had inherited the throne of political administration. Therefore Tsongkhapa says of him, "Miwang Drakpa became famed throughout this domain / As a chieftain dedicated to the Six Yogas tradition."

The first part of the name of the younger brother, Chojey Sonam Gyaltsen, suggests that he was a monk. "Chojey" literally means "Dharma master." Here it is probably being used as an honorific for a monk of aristocratic background. Tsongkhapa's reference to him in the concluding verses of *A Book of Three Inspirations* describes him as one "whose wisdom pulsates / With having read the sacred scriptures in depth, and who / Has become rich in profound spiritual realization." This reinforces the probability that he was a monk.

Bibliography

PART I: TIBETAN TEXTS CITED IN THE INTRODUCTION

A Book of Three Inspirations: A Treatise on the Stages of Training in the Profound Path of Naro's Six Dharmas
    Zab lam na ro'i chos drug gi sgo nas 'khrid pa'i rim pa yid ches gsum ldan zhes bya ba
    by Tsongkhapa the Great (1357-1419)

A Brief Manual on the Manner of Taking Up the Practice of the Stages in Meditation of "Naro's Six Dharmas," Compiled from the Teachings of Jey Rinpochey by Sempa Chenpo Kunzangpa
    Na ro chos drug gi dmigs rim lag tu len tshul bsdus pa rje'i gsungs bzhin sems dpa' chen po kun bzang pas bkod pa
    by Tsongkhapa the Great (1357-1419)

Notes on A Book of Three Inspirations
    Yid ches gsum ldan gyi bshad lung zin bris
    by Jey Sherab Gyatso (1803-1875)

An Ornament for A Book of Three Inspirations
    Na ro chos drug gi zin bris yid ches dgongs rgyan
    by Ngulchu Dharmabhadra (1722-1851)

Prayer to the Lineage Masters of the Six Yogas of Naropa
    Na ro chos drug gi bla brgyud kyi smon lam
    by the Seventh Dalai Lama, Gyalwa Kalzang Gyatso (1708-1757)

A Song in Praise of Tsongkhapa the Great
    rJe Tsong kha pa chen po'i stod pa
    by the Eighth Karmapa, Gyalwa Mikyo Dorjey (1507-1554)

A Source of Every Realization: The Stamp of the Six Yogas of Naropa
   Na ro chos drug gi lag rjes dngos grub kun 'byung
   by Gyalwa Wensapa Lobzang Dondrup (1505-1566)

A Source of Great Ecstasy Realization: A Guide to the Profound Six Yogas of Naropa
   Zab lam na ro'i chos drug gi khrid yig bde chen dngos grub 'byung gnas
   by Nagtsang Tulku (fl. mid-nineteenth c.)

PART II: TEXTS QUOTED BY LAMA TSONGKHAPA

Indian Texts

Titles appear first in English, followed by the abbreviated title used by Tsongkhapa in *A Book of Three Inspirations*. These are followed by the standard longer forms of the titles in Tibetan and Sanskrit, together with the Tibetan canon numbers as they appear in *The Tibetan Tripitaka*, Peking Edition, published in Japan by the Suzuki Research Foundation, 1955-61. Each entry concludes with the Indian author's name; however, texts from the Kangyur (Tib. bKa' 'gyur), all of which are said to be the direct words of the Buddha, are simply listed as "Kangyur."

The Arising of Heruka Tantra
   Tsongkhapa: *He ru ka mngon 'byung*
   Tib. Canon: *dPal khrag 'thung mngon par 'byung ba shes bya ba*
   Skt. *Śrī-heruka-abhyudaya-nāma*
   Peking: 21
   Author: Kangyur

Arising of Samvara Tantra
   Tsongkhapa: *sDom 'byung*
   Tib. Canon: *dPal bde mchog 'byung ba'i rgyud kyi rgyal po chen po*
   Skt. *Śrī-mahāsaṃbarodaya-tantrarāja-nāma*
   Peking: 20
   Author: Kangyur

The Book of Manjushri's Direct Instructions
   Tsongkhapa: *'Jam dpal zhal lung*
   Tib. Canon: *Zhal gyi lung*
   Skt. *Mukhāgama*
   Peking: 2717
   Author: Buddhajñānapāda

The Chakrasamvara Root Tantra
   Tsongkhapa: *bDe mchog rtsa rgyud*
   Tib. Canon: *rGyud kyi rgyal po dpal bde mchog nyung ngu shes bya ba*
   Skt. *Tantrarāja-śrī-laghusambara-nāma*
   Peking: 16
   Author: Kangyur

The Clear Lamp
Tsongkhapa: *sGron gsal*
Tib. Canon: *sGron ma gsal bar byed pa shes bya ba'i rgya che bshad pa*
Skt. *Pradīpoddyotana-nāma-ṭīkā*
Peking: 2650
Author: Candrakīrti

Commentary to the Four Seats Tantra
Tsongkhapa: *gDan bzhi 'grel pa*
Tib. Canon: *rGyud kyi rgyal po dpal gdan bzhi pa'i 'grel pa dran pa'i rgyu mtshan*
Skt. *Śrī-catuḥpīṭha-tantrarājasyaṭīkā-smṛtinibandha-nāma*
Peking: 2478
Author: Bhavabhadra

Compendium of Abhidharma
Tsongkhapa: *Chos kun btus*
Tib. Canon: *Chos mngon pa kun las btus pa shes bya ba*
Skt. *Abhidharma-samuccaya*
Peking: 5550
Author: Asaṅga

Compendium of Tantric Experiences
Tsongkhapa: *sPyod bsdus*
Tib. Canon: *sPyod pa bsdus pa'i sgron ma*
Skt. *Caryā-melāpaka-pradīpa*
Peking: 2668
Author: Āryadeva

Compendium of Wisdom Diamonds
Tsongkhapa: *Ye shes rdo rje kun las btus pa*
Tib. Canon: *Ye shes rdo rje kun las btus pa shes bya ba'i rgyud*
Skt. *Vajrajñāna-samuccaya-nāma-tantra*
Peking: 84
Author: Kangyur

Diamond Rosary Tantra
Tsongkhapa: *rGyud rdo rje phreng ba*
Tib. Canon: *rNal 'byor chen po'i rgyud dpal rdo rje phreng ba mngon par brjod pa rgyud thams cad kyi snying po gsang ba rnam par phye ba shes bya ba*
Skt. *Śrī-vajramāla-abhidhāna-mahāyogatantra-sarvatantrahṛdaya-rahasya-vibhaṅga*
Peking: 82
Author: Kangyur

Diamond Sky Dancer Tantra
Tsongkhapa: *rGyud rdo rje mkha' 'gro*
Tib. Canon: *dPal rdo rje mkha' 'gro bsang ba'i rgyud kyi rgyal po*
Skt. *Śrī-vajraḍākaguhya-tantrarāja*
Peking: 44
Author: Kangyur

Drop of Springtime
Tsongkhapa: *dPyid kyi thig le*
Tib. Canon: *dPyid kyi thig le shes bya ba*
Skt. *Vasanta-tilaka-nāma*
Peking: 2166
Author: Śrī Kṛṣṇa

Elucidation of the Summary of the Five Stages
Tsongkhapa: *Rim lnga rtsa tshig bsdus pa gsal ba*
Tib. Canon: *Rim-pa lnga'i don gsal bar byed pa shes bya ba*
Skt. *Pañcakramārtha-bhāskaraṇa-nāma*
Peking: 2702
Author: Nāgabodhi

The Essential Ornament
Tsongkhapa: *sNying po'i rgyan*
Tib. Canon: *dPal rdo rje snying po rgyan gyi rgyud ces bya ba*
Skt. *Śrī-vajrahṛdayālaṃkāra-tantra-nāma*
Peking: 86
Author: Kangyur

Fifty Verses on the Guru
Tsongkhapa: *Bla ma lnga bcu pa*
Tib. Canon: *Bla ma lnga bcu pa shes bya ba*
Skt. *Guru-pañcāśikā*
Peking: 4544
Author: Aśvaghoṣa

The Five Stages
Tsongkhapa: *Rim lnga*
Tib. Canon: *Rim pa lnga pa shes bya ba*
Skt. *Pañca-krama*
Peking: 2667
Author: Nāgārjuna

The Four Seats Tantra
Tsongkhapa: *gDan bzhi*
Tib. Canon: *dPal gdan bzhi pa'i rnam par bshad pa'i rgyud kyi rgyal po shes bya ba*
Skt. *Śrī-caturpīṭha-vikhyāta-tantrarāja-nāma*
Peking: 69
Author: Kangyur

The Guhyasamaja Tantra
Tsongkhapa: *bSang 'dus rtsa rgyud*
Tib. Canon: *De bzhin gshegs pa thams cad kyi sku gsung thugs kyi gsang ba 'dus pa shes bya ba brtag pa'i rgyal po chen po*
Skt. *Sarvatathāgata-kāya-vākcitta-rahasyo guhyasamāja-nāma-mahākalparāja*
Peking: 81
Author: Kangyur

A Harvest of Oral Tradition Teachings
Tsongkhapa: *Man ngag snye ma*
Tib. Canon: *dPal yang dag par sbyor ba'i rgyud kyi rgyal po'i ryga cher 'grel pa man ngag gi snye ma shes bya ba*
Skt. *Srī-saṃpuṭa-tantrarāja-ṭīkā-āmnāya-mañjarī-nāma*
Peking: 2328
Author: Abhayākaragupta

The Hevajra Root Tantra
See *Hevajra Tantra in Two Sections*

The Hevajra Tantra in Two Sections
Tsongkhapa: *rTags gnyis*
Tib. Canon: *Kye'i rdo rje shes bya ba rgyud kyi rgyal po*
Skt. *He-vajra-tantrarāja-nāma*
Peking: 10
Author: Kangyur

The Lotus Receptacle
Tsongkhapa: *Pad ma can*
Tib. Canon: *Pad ma can shes bya ba'i dka' 'grel* (?)
Skt. *Padmani-nāma-pañjikā* (?)
Peking: 2067 (?)
Author: (?)

The Mark of the Great Seal
Tsongkhapa: *Phyag chen thig le*
Tib. Canon: *dPal phyag rgya chen po'i thig le shes bya ba rnal 'byor ma chen mo'i rgyud kyi rgyal po mnga' bdag*
Skt. *Srī-mahāmudrātilakaṃ-nāma-yoginī-tantrarāja-adhipati*
Peking: 12
Author: Kangyur

The Mystic Kiss Tantra
Tsongkhapa: *Kha sbyor*
Tib. Canon: *rNal 'byor ma bzhi'i kha sbyor gyi rgyud ces bya ba*
Skt. *Catur-yoginī-saṃpuṭa-tantra-nāma*
Peking: 24
Author: Kangyu

The Sambhuta Drop of Springtime
Tsongkhapa: *Sam bhu ta dpyid thig*
Tib. Canon: *dPal kha sbyor thig le shes bya ba rnal 'byor ma'i rgyud kyi rgyal po'i rgya cher 'grel pa yang dag par lta ba'i [d]ran pa'i snang ba shes bya ba*
Skt. *Srī-saṃpuṭa-tilaka-nāma-yoginī-tantrarājasya ṭikā smṛtisaṃdarśanāloka-nāma*
Peking: 2327
Author: Indrabodhi

The Sambhuta Explanatory Tantra
Tsongkhapa: *Sam bhu ta bshad rgyud*
See *A Harvest of Oral Tradition Teachings* above

The Sambhuta Tantra
Tsongkhapa: *Sam bhu ta*
Tib. Canon: *Yang dag par sbyor ba shes bya ba'i rgyud chen po*
Skt. *Samputi-nāma-mahātantra*
Peking: 26
Author: Kangyur

Sixty Stanzas on Emptiness
Tsongkhapa: *Rigs pa drug bcu pa*
Tib. Canon: *Rigs pa drug bcu pa'i tshig le'ur byas ba shes bya ba*
Skt. *Yuktiṣaṣṭikā-kārikā-nāma*
Peking: 5225
Author: Nāgārjuna

Source of Every Siddhi
Tsongkhapa: *dNgos grub kun 'byung*
Tib. Canon: *dNgos grub sgrub pa'i sgo nas sri'u gso ba*
Skt. **Siddhi-sādhanānusāreṇa mṛta-vatsā-cikitsā*
Peking: 3923
Author: Candragomin

Sutra on Entering into the Womb
Tsongkhapa: *mNgal 'jug pa*
Tib. Canon: *'Phags pa tshe dang ldan pa dga' bo mngal du 'jug pa bstan pa shes bya ba theg pa chen po'i mdo*
Skt. *Ārya-āyuṣman-nanda-garbhāvakrānti-nirdésa[-nāma-mahāyāna-sūtra]*
Peking: 760(13)
Author: Kangyur

The Tantra of Interpenetrating Union
Tsongkhapa: *mNyam sbyor*
Tib. Canon: *dPal sang rgyas thams cad dang mnyam par sbyor ba mkha' 'gro sgyu ma bde ba mchog gi rgyud kyi don rnam par bzhad pa shes bya ba*
Skt. *Śrī-sarvabuddha-samayoga-dākinījāla-śambara-tantrārtha-ṭīkā-nāma*
Peking: 2531
Author: Kangyur

Ten Reflections on Simple Suchness
Tsongkhapa: *De kho na nyid bcu pa*
Tib. Canon: *De kho na nyid bcu pa shes bya ba*
Skt. *Tattvadaśaka-nāma*
Peking: 3080
Author: Advayavajra [Maitripa]

Ten Reflections on Simple Suchness: A Commentary
Tsongkhapa: *De kho na nyid bcu pa'i 'grel pa*
Tib. Canon: *De kho na nyid bcu pa'i rgya cher 'grel pa*
Skt. *Tattva-daśaka-ṭīkā*
Peking: 3099
Author: Sahajavajra

Treasury of Abhidharma
Tsongkhapa: *mDzod*
Tib. Canon: *Chos mngon pa'i mdzod kyi tshig le'ur byas pa*
Skt. *Abhidharma-koṣa-kārikā*
Peking: 5590
Author: Vasubandhu

Treatise on Bliss
Tsongkhapa: *dGa' ba'i bstan bcos*
Tib. Canon: *'Dod pa'i bstan bcos shes bya ba*
Skt. *Kāmaśāstra-nāma*
Peking: 3323
Author: Surūpa

Vajra Song of the Six Dharmas
Tsongkhapa: *Chos drug rdo rje'i mgur*
Tib. Canon: *Chos drug gi man ngag shes bya ba*
Skt. *Ṣaḍdharmopadeśa-nāma*
Peking: 4630
Author: Nāropa
Note: Chos drug rdo rje'i mgur *could also refer to Naropa's* Verses on the Whispered Tradition *(Tib.* sNyan rgyud tshig rkang*), which is not found in the Peking Tangyur.*

The Vajra Tent Tantra
Tsongkhapa: *rDo rje mgur*
Tib. Canon: *'Phags pa mkha' 'gro ma rdo rje gur shes bya ba'i rgyud kyi rgyal po chen po'i brtag pa*
Skt. *Ārya-ḍākinī-vajrapañjara-mahātantrarāja-kalpa-nāma*
Peking: 11
Author: Kangyur

The Victorious Nonduality Tantra
Tsongkhapa: *gNyis med rnam rgyal brdzus mo*
Tib. Canon: *dPal de bzhin gshegs pa thams cad kyi gsang ba rnal 'byor chen po rnam par rgyal ba shes bya ba mnyam pa nyid gnyis su med pa'i rgyud kyi rgyal po rdo rje dpal mchog chen po brtag pa dang po*
Skt. *Śrī-sarvatathāgata-guhyatantra-yoga-mahā-rāja-advayasamatā-vijaya-nāma-vajra-śrī-paramamahākalpa-ādi*
Peking: 88
Author: Kangyur

Tibetan Texts

Although Tsongkhapa quotes and refers to numerous Tibetan masters, he mentions only five indigenous Tibetan texts by name. These, together with the names of their authors, are listed below. Tsongkhapa does not provide the textual sources that he used for his numerous quotations from Marpa Lotsawa and Milarepa. However, the verses he ascribes to Marpa exist in a number of sources, including his *Biography* by Tsangpa Rechung. The quotations he ascribes to Milarepa can be found in the *Mila Gurbum* (Tib. *Mi la gur 'bum*), or *Hundred Thousand Songs of Milarepa*.

Eight Instructions in Verse and Prose
   Tib. *Tshig rkang brgyad ma*
   by Marpa Lotsawa

The Early Compendium Root Text
   Tib. *Ka dpe rtsa ba'i sdom snga ma*
   Authorship disputed; probably a compilation by several early Kargyu
      masters

The Later Compendium Root Text
   Tib. *Ka dpe rtsa ba'i sdom phyi ma*
   Authorship disputed; probably a compilation by several early Kargyu
      masters

Treatise on the Four Dharmas
   Tib. *Chos bzhis 'grel pa*
   by Chojey Gampopa

A Verse Guide to the Path
   Tib. *Thabs lam tshigs bcad ma'i lhan thabs*
   by Pal Pakmo Drupa